Cooking With Heart In Mind

A Beginner's Collection Of Nutrient Packed Recipes For A Healthy Heart

Shauve Rivk

Copyright © 2023 by Shauve Rivk

Table of Contents

Introduction

Understanding Heart Health: Navigating the Rythms of Your Cardiovascular Symphony

Importance of a Healthy Heart

Key Nutrients for Cardiovascular Wellness

The Role of Balanced Nutrition

Chapter 1: Kitchen Essentials for Heart Health

Stocking a Heart Healthy Pantry

Choosing the Right Cooking Oils

Essential Tools for Heart-Conscious

Cooking

Chapter 2: Breakfasts to Jumpstart your

Health

Energizing Smoothie Bowls

Whole Grain Morning Muffins

Heart-Healthy Oatmeal Variations

Chapter 3: Lunches for Sustained Vitality

Colorful Quinoa Salad with Fresh

Vegetables

Grilled Chicken and Avocado Wraps

Lentil Soup for Heartwarming Nutrition

Chapter 4: Dinner Delights for Cardiovascular Wellness

Lemon and Dill Baked Salmon

Quinoa and Vegetable Stir-Fry with a

Quinoa and Vegetable Stir-Fry

Stuffed Bell Peppers with Turkey and Brown Rice

Lentil and Sweet Potato

Grilled Chicken with Quinoa Salad

Tomato and Basil Whole Grain Pasta

Skillet with Chickpeas and Spinach

Baked Salmon with Lemon-Dill Sauce

Veggie-Packed Stir-Fry with Tofu

Veggie-Packed Stir-Fry Harmony: Tofu with Protein

Quinoa and Black Bean Stuffed Peppers

Quinoa and Black Bean Stuffed Peppers

Fiesta:Protein-Rich Quinoa

Chapter 5: Snacks for Heart-Smart Munching

Roasted Chickpeas, Crunchy

Dark Chocolate Nutty Trail Mix

Greek Yogurt and Berries Parfait

Hummus-Dipped Veggie Sticks

Kale Chips Baked Taste

Almond Butter Apple Slices

Avocado Toast on Whole Wheat Bread

Smoothie with Berries and Chia Seeds

Roasted Chickpeas with Herbs

Nut and Seed Trail Mix

Almonds and Walnuts

Dark Chocolate Delectable

Dried Fruits with Chew

Berry Chia Seed Pudding

Vanilla Extract Almond Flour Banana Bread

Heartwarming Oatmeal Raisin Cookies

Fruits and Vegetables Sorbet

Wholesome Carrot Cake Bites

Grilled Pineapple with Honey and Mint

Dark Chocolate and Berry Clusters

Medley of Mixed Berries

Crunchy Nut Combination

Heart-Healthy Banana Bread

Berry Bliss Smoothie Popsicles

Popsicle Sticks and Molds

Chapter 6: Beverages That Love Your Heart

Hibiscus Berry Iced Tea

Cubes of Ice Citrus-Infused Water

Green Tea with Lemon and Ginger

Berry-Beet Smoothie

Minty Cucumber Cooler

Golden Turmeric Latte

Pomegranate Green Tea Smoothie

Refreshing Green Tea Lemonade

Lemonade Green Tea

Antioxidant-Packed Berry Smoothie

Watermelon Rose Refresher

Ginger Lemon Zest

Chapter 7: Mindful Eating Habits for Heart Health

Accepting Nutrient-Dense Options

Mindful Hydration

Mindful Eating and Gratitude

Portion Control and Balance

The Visual Guide to Understanding Portion Control

Smart Substitutions for Heart-Healthy Cooking

Eating with Awareness and Gratitude

Conclusion

Nutritional Information for Select Recipes

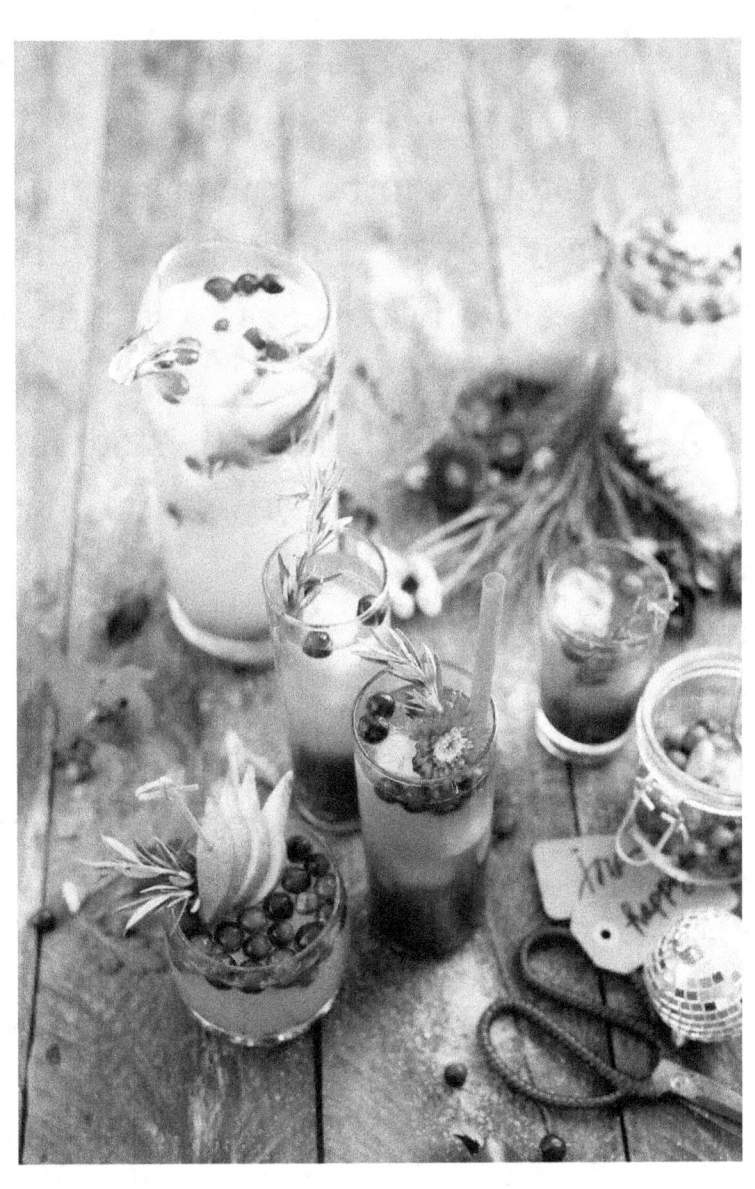

Introduction

This cookbook is your partner on a journey to radiant well-being in the delicate art of producing foods that love your heart back. Allow the pages that follow to be your passport to a world in which the kitchen is not only a creative area but also a sanctuary where every item is carefully picked to support the rhythm of your cardiovascular health.

We'll dig into the subtleties of heart health, studying not only the science behind it but also the culinary poetry that can convert your meals into a chorus of well-being.

You'll learn about the essentials of a heart-healthy kitchen, from pantry staples to cooking oils that bring out the best in your food. This book will encourage you to indulge in morning rituals that launch your day with heart-healthy enthusiasm as the sun rises on your gourmet trip.

From colorful smoothie bowls to whole-grain muffins that promise long-lasting energy, your breakfast table becomes a canvas for sustenance and enjoyment.

Midday and evening are great periods for heart-healthy meals. Learn how to prepare salads that explode with nutrients, wraps that dance with flavors, and meals that are both elegant and healthful. With salmon, tofu stir-fries, and stuffed peppers on the menu, the dinner table morphs into a paradise where every meal is a step toward cardiovascular health. Allow the kitchen to become a stage where your heart takes center stage and each ingredient plays a supporting role in the drama that is your well-being.

So, tie your apron, polish your knives, and join me on this culinary trip where deliciousness and heart health combine in a celebration of life, love, and the art of heart-healthy cooking.

Understanding Heart Health: Navigating the Rythms of Your Cardiovascular Symphony

The heart is the conductor in the rich fabric of our bodies, leading the symphony of life. Understanding heart health is more than simply understanding medical lingo; it is an investigation of the throbbing life that nourishes us. As we move through this book, consider your heart not merely as an organ but also as the focal center of your health—a rhythmic dance that demands knowledge and care. The symphony of the heart is the rhythm of your existence, a harmonic pulse that keeps every cell, organ, and instant of your life alive. The Cardiovascular

Wellness includes understanding the combination of lifestyle, genetics, and environmental factors. It's a delicate ballet in which diet, exercise, and stress management all have an influence on the heartbeat. As we dive into the intricacy, see your heart as part of a vast ballet in which every movement counts. The vitality of the heart is intimately connected to the nutrients it receives. Uncover the relevance of omega-3 fatty acids, antioxidants, and fiber—nutritional notes that add to a harmony of cardiovascular fitness. Allow your plate to become a painting with the brilliant colors of fruits, veggies, and nutritious grains that rejuvenate your heart with every mouthful. Establishing a harmonic balance is crucial in heart health investigations. Learn how to maintain good blood pressure, cholesterol levels, and general cardiovascular fitness. Learn to fine-tune your lifestyle like a professional composer to guarantee that the heart's symphony sounds in perfect harmony. The rate of physical exertion is intrinsically tied to the beat of the heart. Immerse yourself in the joy of movement, understanding how exercise not only increases but also improves the efficiency of the heart muscle. Whether it's the dance of a brisk promenade or the intensity of cardiovascular exercises, each step adds to your heart's health score. Learn how to mute the discordant tones and restore harmony with mindfulness techniques and the healing power of calm. Navigate the diverse tempos of youth to senior years, modifying your lifestyle and behaviors to fit your heart's growing requirements. Celebrate the persistent symphony that has followed you through every stage of life.

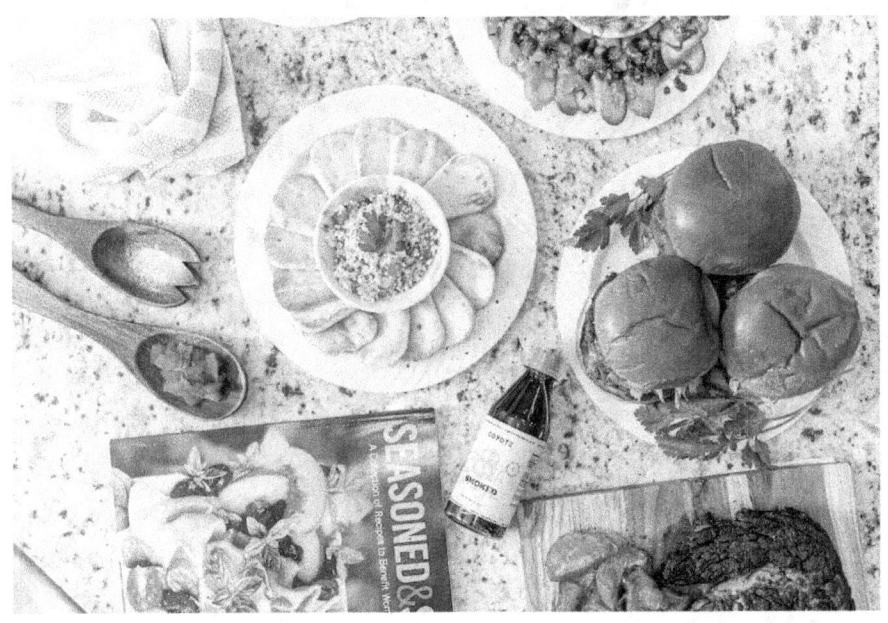

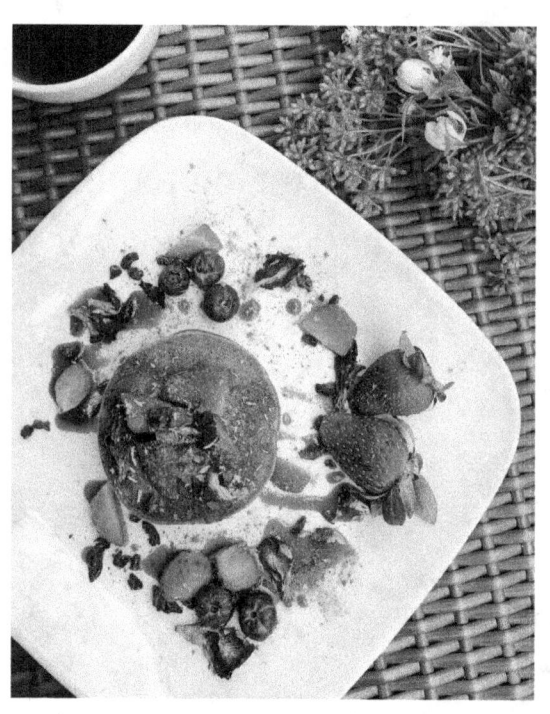

Importance of a Healthy Heart

The heart emerges as the constant protagonist in the tough play of life, throbbing in regular coordination to preserve the symphony of our existence. The value of a healthy heart extends beyond the limits of basic anatomy; it is the hub of energy, Consider your heart to be a sentinel, keeping watch at the crossroads of life and death. Every beat is a proclamation, a tribute to its relentless struggle to sustain the constant rhythm of existence. The significance of a healthy heart arises from its position as the conductor of a symphony that plays from the time we take our first breath until the last exhale. The heart is more than simply a muscle; it is a lifeline, transporting oxygen and nutrients to every area of our body. Its value is founded on its capacity to nurture and guarantee that every cell survives in the presence of life-sustaining materials. This lifeline frays without a healthy heart, and the very essence of energy starts to fade. A healthy heart appears as the valiant guardian against the maelstrom of illnesses in the theater of health. It stands firm, warding off the shadows of cardiovascular disorders that lurk in the shadows of our contemporary lives. Its relevance goes beyond the individual, functioning as a beacon of hope for families, communities, and civilizations at large. A healthy heart is more than simply a passive spectator; it is also an active participant in the behaviors that define us. It ignites the flames of endurance and strength, enabling us to climb mountains, cross valleys, and enjoy the boundless possibilities of an active existence. Its relevance arises from its capacity to act as both the motor and the fuel for our bodily pursuits. Beyond the physical, the heart is the emotional conductor of our existence. It flutters with delight, quickens with enthusiasm, and weeps with sadness. A healthy heart fosters not only physical well-being but also emotional resilience, helping us to manage life's various obstacles with grace and tenacity. Imagine a fountain of life and energy, and you'll discover the heart at its source. A healthy heart is like a spring that never runs dry, supplying the strength required to embrace each day with excitement. It pulls us ahead, reminding us that life is a journey designed to be taken in stride. A healthy heart resonates across time in the broad fabric of generations, leaving an everlasting impression on the heritage we inherit. Its value stretches beyond our own lifetime, echoing as a gift to those who come after—a monument to a life well-lived and a heart well-cared for.

Key Nutrients for Cardiovascular Wellness

Nutrition is the primary dancer in the gourmet ballet of heart health, with each nutrient a coordinated movement that contributes to the symphony of cardiovascular wellbeing. Let us embark on a voyage through the key nutrients, finding the bright palette that nourishes and fortifies the heart.

1. **Omega-3 Fatty Acids:** Consider omega-3 fatty acids to be the fluid, beautiful motions of the heart's dance. These important fatty acids, which are high in fatty fish such as salmon, mackerel, and flaxseeds, act synergistically to decrease inflammation, lower blood pressure, and promote blood vessel flexibility. Consider them the nectar that keeps the cardiovascular system working smoothly.

2. **Antioxidants:** Antioxidants are the heart's symphony's alert protectors. They are plentiful in colored fruits and vegetables and help to neutralize free radicals, reducing oxidative stress, which may damage arteries and risk heart health. Antioxidants, which may be found in everything from colorful berries to leafy greens, constitute an essential ensemble that protects the heart from the ravages of aging.

3. **Fiber:** fiber is the ebb and flow of the digestive dance. Fiber, which is rich in whole grains, fruits, and legumes, not only promotes digestion but also helps decrease cholesterol levels. The digestive dance maintains the heart's rhythm, which is harmonic and unobstructed, by keeping a regular speed.

4. **Potassium**: potassium is the conductor that guides the flow of electrolytes in the heart's performance. Potassium, which is rich in bananas, sweet potatoes, and leafy greens, helps moderate blood pressure by lowering salt levels. It ensures that the electrical impulses of the heart conduct freely, resulting in a steady and well-regulated beat.

5. **Magnesium:** magnesium is the relaxing intermission in the composition of the heart. Magnesium, which is present in nuts, seeds, and leafy greens, promotes muscular relaxation, especially the crucial relaxing of the heart muscle. It assists in the preservation of appropriate blood pressure and rhythm, giving a calming pause in the heart's constant symphony.

6. **Vitamin K** is the calcium director. It is the director, guiding calcium to its designated duties in the heart's function. Vitamin K, which is plentiful in dark, leafy greens, assures that calcium accumulates in bones rather than arteries, limiting arterial calcification and adding to overall heart health. In the calcium dance, it's the exact choreographer.

7. **Vitamin D:** vitamin D is a conductor, bringing out the sun's rays to accomplish their work. Vitamin D, which is generated in the skin when exposed to sunshine and contained in fatty fish, enhances heart health by supporting overall circulatory function. It is crucial for calcium absorption, which is needed for robust and healthy hearts.

8. **B Vitamins:** are the metabolic choreographers who keep the metabolism operating smoothly and effectively. B vitamins such as B6, B12, and folic acid, which are found in nutritious grains, lean meats, and green leafy vegetables, assist in the breakdown of homocysteine, a chemical associated with cardiovascular disease. They maintain the metabolic cycle in rhythm, which supports heart health. Let each vitamin be a note in the heart's symphony—a dazzling, significant component that adds to the overall harmony of cardiovascular well-being—in this investigation of key nutrients for cardiovascular health. By integrating these nutrients into your diet, you help your heart continue its delicate dance through the rhythms of life.

The Role of Balanced Nutrition

A balanced diet takes center stage as the choreographer in the difficult dance of health, ensuring that every vitamin and every calorie contribute to the symphony of well-being. Consider balanced food to be the guiding force that orchestrates a harmonic dance between key ingredients, resulting in a robust and healthy cardiovascular composition.

1. **The Energy Connection:** A nutritious diet is the fuel that runs the heart's engine.

A balanced diet of macronutrients—carbohydrates, proteins, and fats—is vital for the heart, just as it is for a vehicle. Carbohydrates offer quick energy, proteins repair and build tissues, and excellent fats provide long-term energy and cardiovascular health.

2. **The Nutrient Ensemble for Cardiovascular Health:** a symphony in which each instrument symbolizes a crucial nutrient. A balanced diet ensures that your body obtains a varied assortment of nutrients, including vitamins, minerals,

antioxidants, and fiber. This diversified composition greatly helps cardiovascular health by supporting processes such as blood vessel flexibility, blood pressure management, and overall heart vitality.

3. **Weight Control: The Calorie Dance** The caloric dance is orchestrated by balanced nutrition. It helps regulate weight by creating a harmonic balance between calorie intake and expenditure, which is a key aspect of cardiovascular health. Maintaining a healthy weight decreases the burden on the heart, minimizing the risk of ailments such as hypertension and heart disease.

4. **The Glucose Waltz for Blood Sugar Control:** Allow appropriate eating to be your partner in the glucose waltz. It helps regulate blood sugar levels by regulating carbs, minimizing spikes and crashes that may strain the cardiovascular system. Blood sugar levels that are stable and well-managed contribute to the heart's steady pulse.

5. **Inflammation Reduction:** The anti-inflammatory ballet is choreographed by balanced nutrition. A balanced diet rich in fruits, vegetables, and omega-3 fatty acids helps limit inflammation, which is a crucial element in the development of cardiovascular issues. It generates a pleasant milieu throughout the body, enabling the heart to beat easily.

6. **Cholesterol Management: The Lipid Symphony** Allow appropriate food as the lipid symphony's composer. It helps manage cholesterol levels by supplying heart-healthy fats, soluble fiber, and plant sterols, avoiding plaque accumulation in the arteries. This specific composition guarantees that the blood flow channels stay open and unhindered.

7. **Blood Pressure Control: The Sodium Minuet** The sodium diet is orchestrated by a balanced diet, which carefully manages salt intake to maintain blood pressure. It contributes to the delicate balance that promotes healthy blood pressure by combining potassium-rich foods and eliminating excess salt, lessening the burden on the heart's pumping function. Balanced nutrition encompasses not only what you eat but also how you live. It combines with heart-healthy behaviors such as regular physical exercise, stress management, and appropriate sleep to generate a lifestyle dance that promotes overall cardiovascular health.

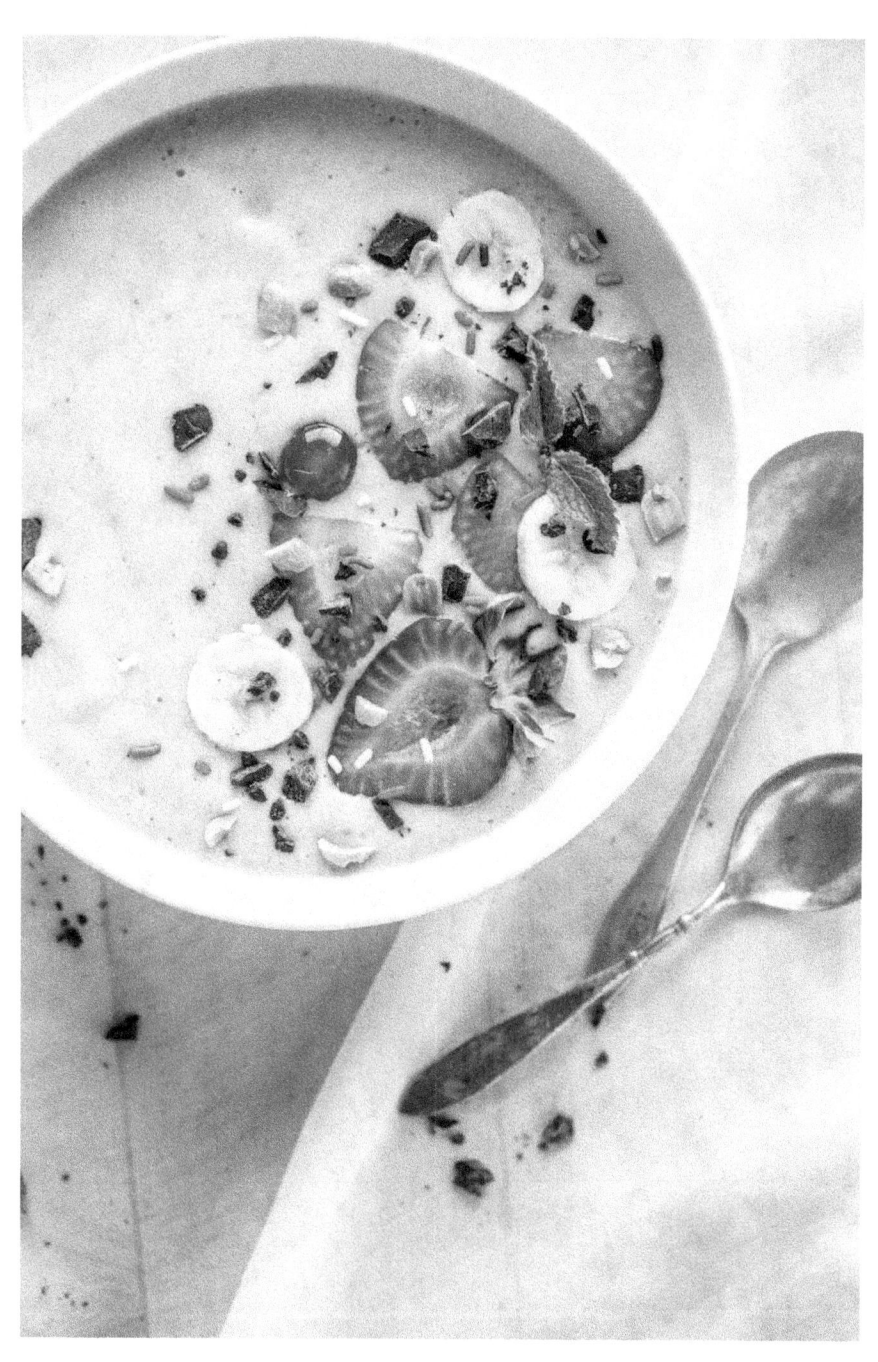

Chapter 1: Kitchen Essentials for Heart Health

Stocking a Heart Healthy Pantry

1. **Whole Grains: The Foundation of the Heart** whole grains are the robust basis of your heart-healthy pantry. Brown rice, quinoa, oats, and whole wheat flour become mainstays, providing a plethora of fiber, vitamins, and minerals. These grains not only enhance cardiovascular health by decreasing cholesterol levels, but they also help you feel motivated throughout the day.

2. **Legumes: Protein-Rich Powerhouses** beans are protein-rich diamonds gracing your cupboard shelves. Beans, lentils, and chickpeas become flexible companions, supplying plant-based protein, fiber, and a range of minerals. Their importance in heart health is based on their capacity to decrease cholesterol, maintain blood sugar levels, and offer a consistent supply of energy without the saturated fats present in certain animal proteins.

3. **Nuts and Seeds: A Hearty Crunch** nuts and seeds are the heart-healthy crunch that adds to the versatility of your cabinet. Almonds, walnuts, chia seeds, and flaxseeds convert into nutritional powerhouses, providing heart-healthy lipids, omega-3 fatty acids, and antioxidants. These nutrients not only promote cardiovascular health but also offer a delightful texture to your food.

4. **Flavorful antioxidants from colorful spices** pick a choice of vivid spices as the great antioxidants that infuse your cupboard with vitality. Turmeric, cinnamon, ginger, and garlic not only add taste to your food, but they also have anti-inflammatory and antioxidant effects. Using the power of these spices enriches your dishes while also boosting your heart health.

5. **Whole Foods: Unprocessed Delight** complete, unprocessed foods are the purest version of your heart-healthy pantry. Choose canned foods with minimal additives and entire fruits and veggies to guarantee that your cupboard is a refuge of pure joy. These selections contain critical vitamins, minerals, and fiber, which boost overall cardiovascular health.

6. **Olive Oil: Liquid Gold for Cardiovascular Health** olive oil is the liquid gold that graces your cupboard shelves. Olive oil, which is abundant in monounsaturated fats and antioxidants, helps heart health by lowering inflammation and decreasing

cholesterol levels. Make it your go-to cooking oil for sautéing, seasoning, and drizzling—it will revolutionize your food in terms of both taste and health.

7. **Whole-Grain Pasta and Brown Rice: Healthier Options** whole-grain pasta and brown rice are healthy alternatives to the carbs in your cupboard. These alternatives provide a complex carbohydrate basis, delivering consistent energy and fiber, which promote digestion and help maintain a healthy weight—an essential component of cardiovascular health.

8. **Plant-Based Proteins:** adding a variety of plant-based proteins to your cupboard, such as tofu, tempeh, and plant-based protein powders are important. These animal protein replacements are not only heart-healthy, but they also contribute to a well-balanced diet that promotes general health. Consider your heart-healthy pantry not just as a storage place but also as the canvas for your culinary creations. Each component is a brushstroke that forms a piece of art about taste and well-being. Allow your pantry to be a reflection of your devotion to robust health and the lovely adventure of heart-conscious living in the heart of your house.

Choosing the Right Cooking Oils

1. **Olive Oil as a Heart Health Elixir** olive oil is the elixir that decorates your culinary canvas. Olive oil is famous for its heart-protective effects owing to its high content of monounsaturated fats and antioxidants. Its capacity to lower inflammation and raise cholesterol levels makes it a crucial component of heart-healthy cooking. Choose extra virgin olive oil for its raw nature, which preserves the most nutrients and taste.

2. **Avocado Oil: A Creamy Delight for Cardiovascular Health** avocado oil is the creamy richness that adds to your heart-healthy arsenal. Avocado oil is a nutrient-rich alternative with a high smoke point and a composition equivalent to olive oil. It includes monounsaturated fats and antioxidants, which boost heart health while delivering a subtle taste that complements a range of cuisines.

3. **Coconut Oil: A Tropical Delight with Heart Advantages** coconut oil is a tropical delicacy that lends a distinctive taste to heart-healthy cooking. While heavy in saturated fats, coconut oil includes medium-chain triglycerides (MCTs), which some studies show may have cardiac benefits. Use it with care, particularly in dishes that may benefit from its peculiar taste.

4. **Canola Oil:** It has a neutral taste and includes heart-healthy fats. Choose canola oil to be a neutral performer that readily adapts to a number of cuisines. Canola oil has a mild taste and a high smoke point. It is rich in heart-healthy monounsaturated fats and low in saturated fats. Its flexibility makes it a great tool in heart-healthy recipes.

5. **Walnut Oil: Nutty Flavors for Heart-Healthy Recipes** walnut oil is the artisanal finishing touch that gives nutty nuances to your culinary creations. Walnut oil, which is abundant in omega-3 fatty acids, antioxidants, and a unique taste, benefits heart health while also boosting the flavor profile of salads, dressings, and drizzles.

6. **Grapeseed Oil: Light and Heart-Healthy** Consider grapeseed oil to be the light, heart-healthy companion in your kitchen symphony. Grapeseed oil includes polyunsaturated fats and vitamin E and has a high smoke point and a moderate taste.

Its adaptability makes it great for sautéing, frying, and baking—a heart-healthy answer for a range of culinary styles.

7. **Flaxseed Oil: An Omega-3 Powerhouse for Cardiovascular Health** flaxseed oil is an omega-3 powerhouse that offers a healthy boost to your culinary repertoire. Flaxseed oil is rich in alpha-linolenic acid (ALA), a plant-based omega-3 fatty acid that improves heart health. To preserve its nutritional worth, use it as a finishing oil in salad dressings or sprinkle it over foods.

8. **Sesame Oil: Nutty Aroma and Cardiovascular Benefits** sesame oil is the fragrant finishing touch that gives nutty nuances to your foods. While it has a unique taste, it adds depth to stir-fries and other Asian-inspired foods. Choose toasted sesame oil for a richer taste, and use it sparingly to reap the advantages of its heart-healthy characteristics.

9. **Sunflower oil** is multipurpose and heart-healthy. Sunflower oil is an adaptable friend that smoothly integrates into heart-healthy cooking. Sunflower oil includes heart-healthy polyunsaturated fats and has a neutral taste and a high smoke point. Its adaptability makes it suited for a broad variety of culinary uses. Look into the adventure of picking the correct cooking oils to be a nuanced investigation of tastes, textures, and, most crucially, heart-friendly possibilities. Allow your

culinary creations to reflect the attention you take in choosing oils that not only enrich the dining experience but also contribute to the symphony of cardiovascular health.

Essential Tools for Heart-Conscious Cooking

Heart-Healthy Cooking Essentials: Step inside your kitchen's pulse, where the tools you chose become instruments of heart-conscious innovation. In this part, we'll look at the essential instruments that may convert your kitchen into a cardiovascular health stage, guaranteeing that every meal is cooked with precision, care, and love.

1. **A High-Quality Chef's Knife** Choose a brilliant chef's knife to be the maestro in command of the symphony of heart-conscious cooking. A well-sharpened, well-balanced knife becomes an extension of your culinary talent, enabling you to slice through fruits, vegetables, and lean meats with ease. With accuracy at your fingertips, you can simply and beautifully create heart-healthy masterpieces.

2. **Cutting Boards:** boards are the firm foundation upon which heart-centered chopping takes place. Choose boards made of

wood or bamboo, which are soft on knife blades and naturally antimicrobial. Allow the rhythmic chopping on these trustworthy surfaces to become a heart-healthy dance in your kitchen routine.

3. **The Smooth Operator for Heart-Healthy Smoothies: A High-Quality Blender** Choose a high-quality blender as the smooth operator that converts fruits and vegetables into heart-healthy elixirs. Whether you're preparing nutrient-dense smoothies or silky soups, a trustworthy blender guarantees that the fiber and nutritious value of your components are kept, adding to your cardiovascular health.

4. **Nonstick Cookware: Easy Heart-Healthy Saute** Consider nonstick cookware to be the most handy instrument for heart-healthy sautéing. These pans limit the danger of excessive fats in your meals by using less oil. Choose high-quality, PFOA-free choices to guarantee that your heart-healthy cooking is not damaged by dangerous ingredients.

5. **The Steamer Basket: A Gentle Approach to Heart-Healthy Cooking** Choose a steamer basket as a reasonable way to cook heart-healthy food. This device helps you maintain the nutritional content of your veggies while avoiding the need for added fats. The steam dance grows into a

heart-conscious method, conserving tastes and nutrients in every meal.

6. **Crispy Indulgence with Heart-Healthy Precision** Consider an air fryer to be a crispy pleasure that is also heart-healthy. This multipurpose gadget utilizes hot air to generate a crispy surface without using much oil, making it a healthier alternative to deep-frying. Enjoy the delightful pleasures of your favorite recipes while ingesting a fraction of the fat.

7. **Salad Spinner: The Art of Crisp Greens in Motion** Focus on a salad spinner to have the spinning expertise that keeps your greens fresh and ready for substantial salads. Removing extra moisture helps dressings adhere more readily while protecting the freshness of your leafy greens. Allow your salads' rich colors and textures to become a celebration of cardiovascular health.

8. **Measuring Instruments: A Symphony of Precise Portions** Consider measuring spoons to be a symphony of exact proportions in heart-healthy cooking. Accurate measurements guarantee that you adequately balance your components while maintaining heart-healthy serving proportions. From measuring cups to kitchen scales, these tools become your partners in the preparation of delicious, heart-healthy meals.

9. **Food Processor: The Multitasking Virtuoso of Heart-Healthy Recipes** Consider a food processor to be a

dynamic maestro that easily converts materials into heart-healthy masterpieces. A food processor adds a layer of creativity to your heart-healthy kitchen, from chopping and pureeing to producing nutrient-rich nut butters. Accept its adaptability to create a symphony of sensations and experiences. As you fill your kitchen with these vital tools, consider each one as a companion on your road to cardiovascular health. Allow the pulse of your kitchen to echo the beat of your heart, creating a setting in which accuracy, care, and heart-consciousness interplay in every dish you create.

Chapter 2: Breakfasts to Jumpstart your Health

Energizing Smoothie Bowls: These bowls, overflowing with brilliant colors and minerals, serve as a canvas for both art and nourishment. Blend a symphony of fruits, greens, and superfoods, then top with heart-healthy delights like almonds, seeds, and honey.

Whole Grain Muffins: A Sweet Start to the Day These muffins give constant energy and nutritional fiber as they are prepared with whole wheat flour, oats, and other healthy ingredients.

Add nutrient-dense ingredients like berries, almonds, or seeds to build a morning symphony that will delight your palette and feed your heart.

Overnight Oats: A Prelude to Heart-Healthy Nutrition Combining oats with yogurt or milk and soaking them overnight results in a nutrient-dense meal that takes little effort. Make your bowls your own by adding fruits, nuts, and a touch of sweetness to transform your morning into a harmonic hymn to cardiovascular health.

Avocado Toasts with Nutrients: A Heart-Healthy Composition Spread creamy avocado over whole grain bread and top with tomatoes, poached eggs, or seeds to add layers of flavor. These toasts blend healthy fats, fiber, and a rainbow of vitamins and minerals to create a delicious miracle.

Greek Yogurt Parfaits: Heart-Healthy Layers of Indulgence To make a parfait that balances textures and tastes, mix creamy Greek yogurt with fresh fruits, granola, and a drizzle of honey. This meal provides a fantastic symphony for your taste sensations and your heart because it is packed with protein, probiotics, and antioxidants.

Chia Seed Puddings: Heart-Healthy Treats These delectable meals mix chia seeds with milk or plant-based substitutes to achieve a pudding-like consistency overnight. For a morning treat rich in omega-3 fatty acids, fiber, and critical minerals, top with fruits, nuts, or a dollop of yogurt.

Savory Elegance for Heart-Healthy Mornings: Veggie Omelets Vegetable omelets are a beautiful elegance that will brighten your heart-healthy mornings. For a nutrient-dense breakfast, mix eggs with a choice of bright veggies, herbs, and a sprinkling of cheese. This delectable delicacy's protein and fiber make for a delightful and heart-healthy start to your day.

Whole Grain Pancakes: Fluffy Layers of Heart-Healthy Delight Choose whole-grain pancakes as your fluffy mounds of heart-healthy delight. When cooked with whole wheat flour or oats, these pancakes become a blank canvas for your ideas. Top with fresh fruits, yogurt, or a drizzle of pure maple syrup for a balanced morning delight with a touch of joy.

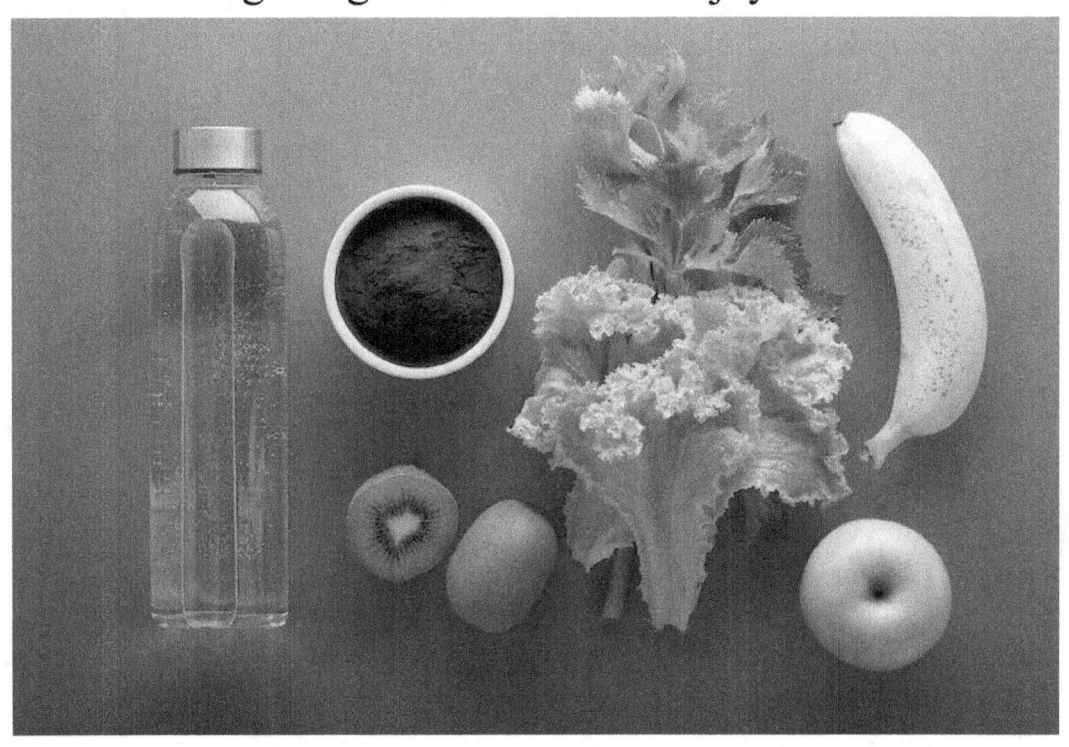

Energizing Smoothie Bowls

Start your day with an exciting smoothie bowl—a symphony of colors, flavors, and nutrients that will get your heart racing. In this part, we'll look at the artistry of crafting these beneficial and beautifully appealing bowls that become a celebration of heart-healthy living.

1. **The Canvas: A Variety of Nutrient-Dense Fruits** Choose the foundation of your invigorating smoothie bowl to be a canvas painted with a rainbow of nutrient-rich fruits. Blend together berries, bananas, mangoes, or other fruits of your choosing. These fruits are not only rich in vitamins and antioxidants, but they also add natural sweetness and brilliant colors to your morning creation.

2. **Greek Yogurt or Plant-Based Alternatives for the Body** Consider your smoothie bowl's body as a picture that cradles the brightness of fruits. Greek yogurt, with its creamy texture and high protein content, is a fantastic option. Choose almond, coconut, or soy yogurt for a plant-based option with a creamy foundation that enhances the fruity symphony.

3. **The Boost: Superfoods for Increased Nutritional Abilities** For omega-3 fatty acids and fiber, add a teaspoon of chia seeds,

flaxseeds, or hemp seeds. Spirulina, a green superfood, provides antioxidants, vitamins, and minerals, converting your smoothie bowl into a nutritious powerhouse.

4. **Honey or maple syrup as a sweetener** To add natural sweetness, sprinkle with honey or pure maple syrup. These sweeteners not only have a nice flavor, but they also deliver extra antioxidants and may have anti-inflammatory qualities.

5. **Nuts, seeds, or granola for crunch** For heart-healthy fats and texture, top your creation with a handful of nuts—almonds, walnuts, or pistachios. Alternatively, for a wonderful crunch, add chia seeds, pumpkin seeds, or a modest bit of granola.

6. **The Artistic Finish: Fresh Fruits and Berries Sliced** Make a beautiful arrangement of kiwi slices, strawberries, blueberries, or other seasonal fruits. This not only increases the visual attractiveness but also delivers a diversity of textures and tastes in each mouthful.

7. **Add a dash of greens for a heart-healthy twist.** Spinach or kale combines beautifully with the fruity combination, giving vitamins, minerals, and antioxidants. Because of the moderate taste, the greens complement rather than overshadow the whole flavor.

8. **Enjoy your morning ritual mindfully.** Take a seat, take each mouthful, and appreciate the symphony of flavors and

sensations. Allow your morning routine to be a celebration of nutrition, setting the tone for the remainder of your heart-healthy day. Allow each ingredient in your refreshing smoothie bowls to be a note in the song of a heart-healthy meal. This bowl is more than just a meal; it's a creative expression, a burst of energy, and a devotion to nurturing your heart and well-being from the get-go.

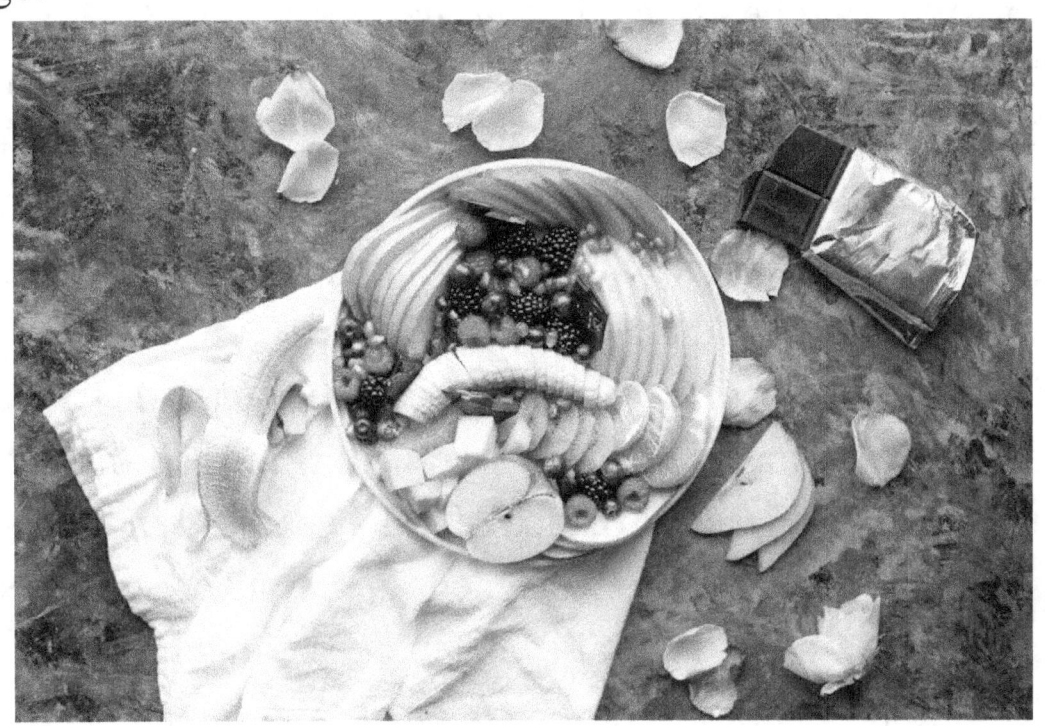

Whole Grain Morning Muffins

Start your day with whole-grain muffins, a delectable blend of nutritious components that not only start your day but also care for your heart's well-being. In this part, we'll look at how to prepare these nutrient-dense muffins that perfectly integrate taste, texture, and heart-healthy alternatives.

1. **Whole wheat flour or oatmeal as the foundation** These fiber-rich options give a firm foundation for your muffins, providing a continuous flow of energy and increasing heart health. Whole grains are abundant in critical elements such as vitamins, minerals, and antioxidants.

2. **Fruits and natural sweeteners give natural sweetness** Think of the natural sweetness in your muffins as a light touch that improves their taste. To add natural sweetness and moisture, add mashed bananas, unsweetened applesauce, or shredded carrots. Alternatively, natural sweeteners such as honey or pure maple syrup give a mild sweetness without sacrificing heart-healthy alternatives.

3. **Nuts and seeds are rich in heart-healthy fats** Add a handful of chopped nuts—walnuts, almonds, or pecans—for an omega-3 fatty acid boost and a pleasant crunch. Sprinkle chia seeds or

flaxseeds on top to increase the nutritional profile with fiber and healthy fats.

4. **Greek Yogurt or Plant-Based Alternatives for Protein** Greek yogurt offers a creamy mouthfeel as well as a protein punch. If you wish to go plant-based, use almond or soy yogurt to preserve the richness and protein content.

5. **Fiber-Rich Supplement: Dried Fruits or Berries** Add dried fruits like raisins, cranberries, or chopped dates for a terrific flavor and fiber boost. Fresh berries, such as blueberries or raspberries, are very tasty and rich in antioxidants.

6. **Aromatic Elements: Vanilla Extract or Spices** For a beautiful and calming undertone, add a teaspoon of pure vanilla essence. Spices like cinnamon, nutmeg, or cardamom, on the other hand, will infuse your muffins with warm, pleasant fragrances and an extra layer of heart-healthy delight.

7. **Baking Powder or Baking Soda as a Rising Agent** To give bread a nice rise and fluffy texture, add baking powder or baking soda. These leavening ingredients produce a fine crumb while enabling you to adjust the quantity of salt in your heart-healthy creation.

8. **Garnish with oats or nuts for a heartfelt presentation** Top the muffins with a sprinkle of oats or a few additional chopped

nuts. This not only improves the look but also adds a wonderful crunch. Turn each muffin into a piece of heart-conscious art.

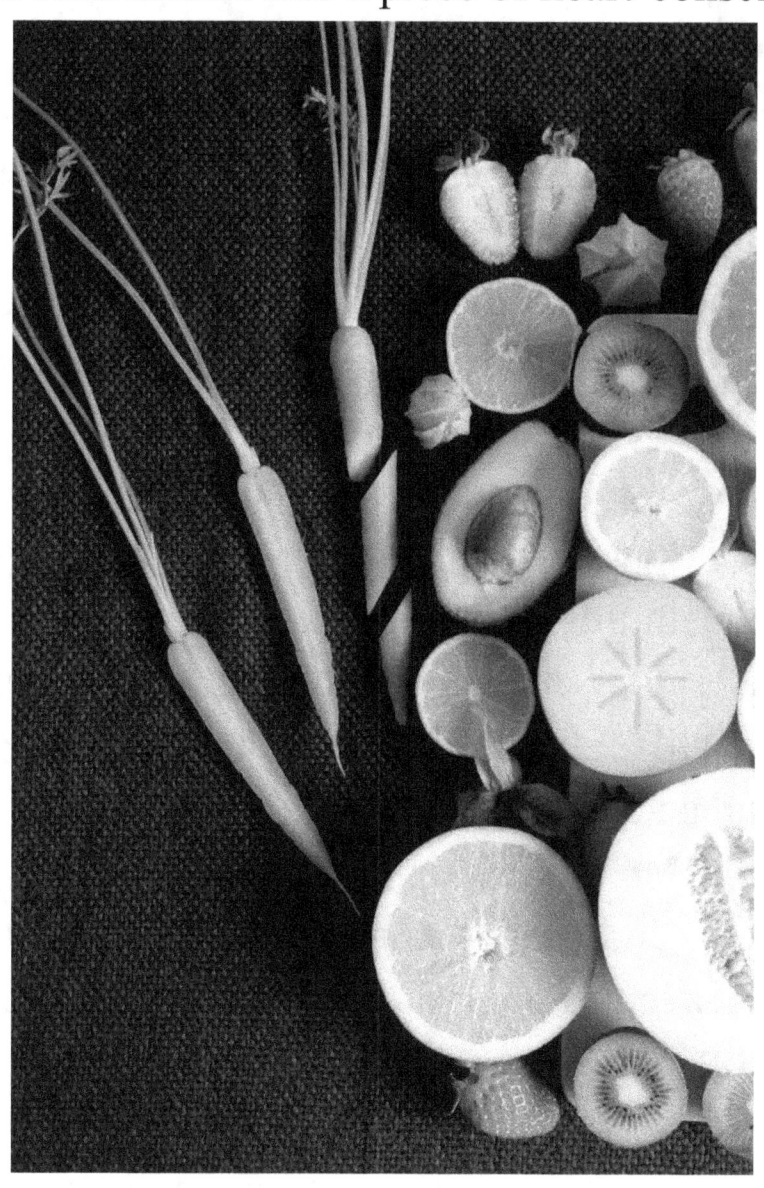

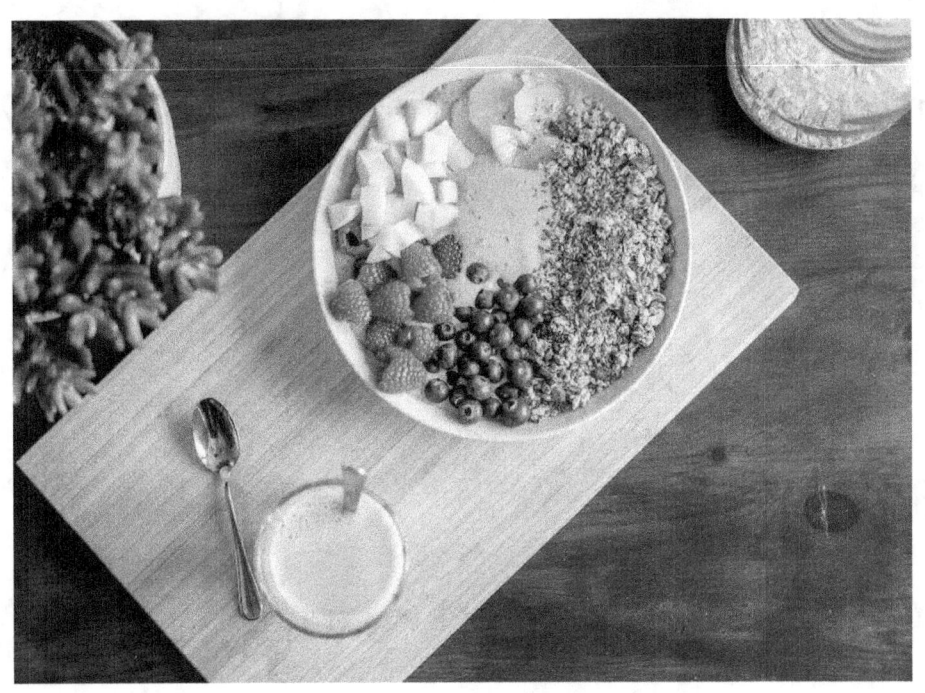

Heart-Healthy Oatmeal Variations

Step into the heart-healthy world of oatmeal variants, a canvas of nutritional alternatives that showcase the warmth and wholesomeness of oats. In this part, we'll look at a selection of inventive and heart-healthy oatmeal dishes, each of which delivers a symphony of tastes, textures, and nutritional advantages.

1. **Traditional Nut and Berry Oatmeal Bowl** A heart-healthy version that blends the soothing warmth of oats with the crunch

of almonds or walnuts. This invention not only thrills your taste buds, but it also supplies the minerals and antioxidants you need to start your day.

Ingredients:
1 pound of rolled oats
1 cup water or milk (dairy or vegan)
1 tablespoon almonds or walnuts, chopped
1/2 cup berries, mixed
Optional sprinkle of honey or maple syrup

2. **Oatmeal with Apple Cinnamon Walnuts** This version not only brings comfort to your morning ritual, but it also includes a nutritious combination of fiber, vitamins, and omega-3 fatty acids.

Ingredients:
1 pound of rolled oats
1 cup water or milk (dairy or vegan)
1/2 diced apple
1/2 teaspoon cinnamon powder
1 tbsp. chopped walnuts
Optional sprinkle of honey or maple syrup

3. **Oatmeal Bowl with Tropical Paradise** This tropical delicacy not only transports your taste sensations, but it also includes a range of heart-healthy minerals.

Ingredients:
1 pound of rolled oats
1 cup of water or coconut milk
1/4 cup pineapple, chopped
1 tbsp. shredded coconut
1 tbsp. macadamia nuts, chopped, and a lime zest

4. **Overnight Oats with Chia Seeds and Mixed Berries** This offers a delicious combination of tastes as well as the additional benefit of omega-3 fatty acids from chia seeds. The overnight preparation offers a stress-free and heart-healthy start to your day.

Ingredients:
1 pound of rolled oats
1/2 cup milk (dairy or vegan)
1 tbsp. chia seeds

1/2 cup berries, mixed

Optional sprinkle of honey or maple syrup

5. **Elegance Pumpkin Spice Pecan Oatmeal** This seasonal delight not only calms you but also nourishes your body with a number of critical nutrients.

Ingredients:

1 pound of rolled oats

1 cup water or milk (dairy or vegan)

2 teaspoons pureed canned pumpkin

1 teaspoon pumpkin spice combination

1 tbsp. chopped pecans Optional sprinkle of honey or maple syrup

6. **Oatmeal with Savory Spinach and Feta** This delicious dish blends nutrient-dense spinach with the satiating richness of feta cheese to produce a breakfast choice that is both enjoyable and beneficial.

Ingredients:

1 pound of rolled oats

1 cup veggie broth (or water) a couple fresh spinach leaves

1 tablespoon feta cheese, crumbled
Season with salt and pepper to taste.

7. Chocolate Indulgence in Banana Almond Butter Oatmeal

This exquisite combination is a symphony of rich tastes and heart-conscious pleasures that will offer you a terrific start to your day.

Ingredients:

1 pound rolled oats;
1 cup milk (dairy or vegan)
1 teaspoon cocoa powder
1/2 mashed banana
1 tbsp. almond butter
Optional sprinkle of honey or maple syrup

Let each bowl of these heart-healthy oatmeal varieties be a celebration of taste, nutrition, and the dedication to supporting your heart with every great mouthful.

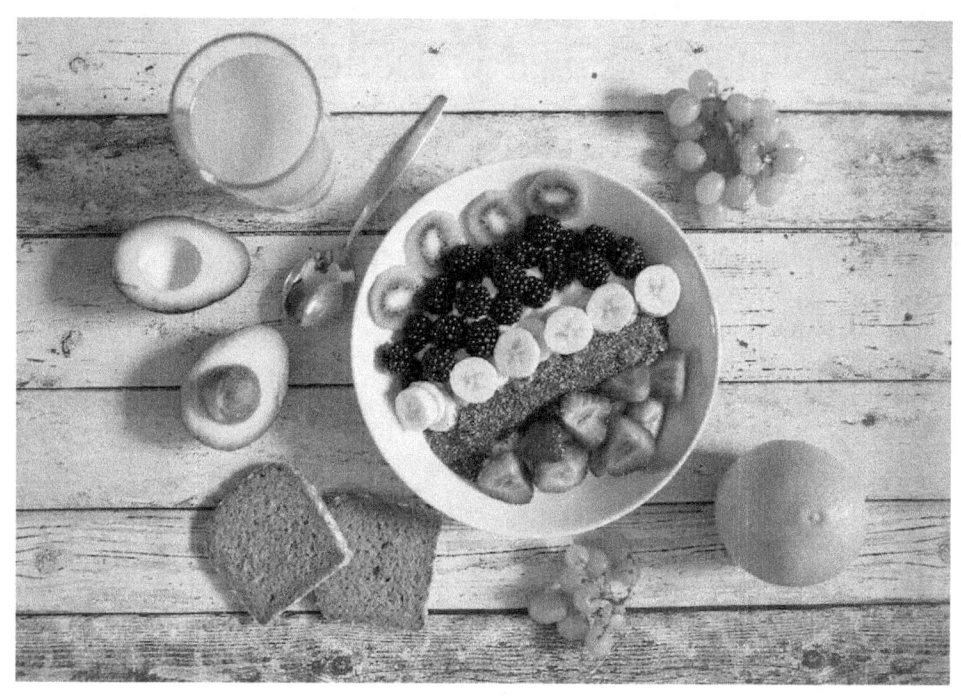

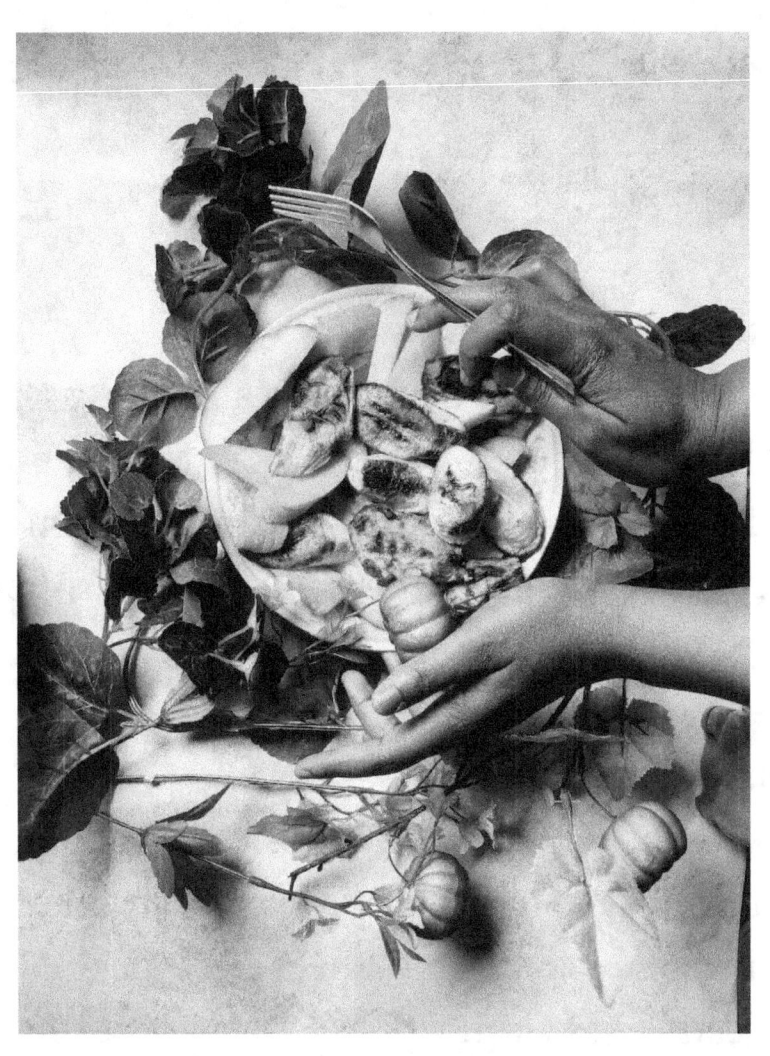

Chapter 3: Lunches for Sustained Vitality

Power Quinoa and Veggie Bowl

As the focus of your heart-healthy meal, try a gorgeous quinoa and vegetable power bowl. This meal is a symphony of tastes, textures, and necessary minerals, with protein from quinoa and a variety of colorful veggies. For an extra heart-healthy touch, drizzle with olive oil and sprinkle with feta cheese.

Ingredients:

1 cup quinoa, cooked Vegetables: various (bell peppers, cherry tomatoes, cucumber) Herbs of Provence (parsley or cilantro) Dressing with olive oil Feta cheese, if desired Salad with Salmon, Avocado, and Citrus

Consider a delectable salmon and avocado citrus salad—a light but satisfying meal that blends heart-healthy omega-3 fatty acids with a blast of citrus brightness. The combination of grilled salmon, creamy avocado, and a zesty citrus vinaigrette provides a symphony of tastes that will feed your body while also satisfying your taste buds.

Ingredients: Fillets of grilled salmon Greens (spinach, arugula, or watercress).
Mix Avocado slices Dressing and citrus vinaigrette
Optional pomegranate seeds

Lentil and Vegetable This stew, which is strong in plant-based protein, fiber, and a variety of vegetables, not only delivers constant energy but also benefits heart health. Serve with whole-grain bread for a balanced and heart-healthy lunch.

Ingredients:
1 pound of lentils Vegetables (carrots, celery, onions, and tomatoes)
Broth of veggies Herbs and garlic for flavor
Optional whole-grain bread

Stuffed Peppers with Turkey and Quinoa Choose vibrant bell peppers stuffed with a combination of lean turkey and quinoa for a protein-packed lunch that balances delectable ingredients with heart-healthy options. The peppers not only offer color but also crucial vitamins and antioxidants, supporting overall cardiovascular health.

Ingredients:
Cayenne peppers
Ground turkey that is lean
Quinoa with tomato sauce
Seasoning herbs and spices

Wrapped Chickpea and Spinach Salad This wrap gives a burst of freshness and taste while being filled with plant-based protein, fiber, and a variety of veggies. For an extra heart-healthy touch, wrap it in a whole-grain or spinach wrap.

Ingredients:
Chickpeas, cleaned and drained spinach leaves, fresh Wrap Greek yogurt dressing over cherry tomatoes, diced cucumber, sliced whole grain, or spinach.

Bowl of Quinoa and Black Beans with Avocado This breakfast not only satisfies your appetite but also offers a nutrient-rich foundation for lasting energy throughout the day.

Ingredients: Quinoa has been cooked. Avocado, chopped salsa or pico de gallo, and black beans, canned and drained, garnished with lime wedges

Stir-Fry with Grilled Chicken and Vegetables Stir-frying retains the nutritional content of the ingredients while infusing the meal with a heart-healthy taste.

Ingredients: thinly sliced chicken breast
Vegetable stir-fry (broccoli, bell peppers, and snap peas)
To taste, add soy sauce or teriyaki sauce.
Serve with brown rice or quinoa.

Salad with Quinoa from the Mediterranean This salad, filled with bright veggies, olives, and feta cheese, delivers a great mix of flavor and nutritional advantages.

Ingredients: Quinoa cooked, cucumber halved, Kalamata olives diced, Feta cheese sliced, and lemon vinaigrette dressing crumbled.

Colorful Quinoa Salad with Fresh Vegetables

Colorful Quinoa Salad—a healthy and visually stunning salad that blends the nutritional richness of quinoa with a mix of fresh vegetables—will thrill your senses. This heart-healthy meal not only excites your taste sensations but also gives you a blast of nutrients and colors to help you get through the day.

Ingredients:

1 cup of rinsed and cooked quinoa

1 cup cherry tomatoes, halved

1 cup cucumber, diced 1/2 cup red bell pepper, diced

1/2 cup yellow bell pepper, diced

1/4 cup red onion, coarsely chopped

1/4 cup fresh cilantro or parsley, crushed

Optional: 1/4 cup chopped Kalamata olives

To create the dressing:

3 tbsp. extra virgin olive oil

1 tbsp. balsamic vinegar

1 minced garlic clove

1 tsp. Dijon mustard Season with salt and pepper to taste.

Instructions:

Rinse 1 cup of quinoa in cold water and cook it according to package directions.

Allow it to cool to room temperature after cooking.

Make the vegetables: Cut the cherry tomatoes in half. Cucumber, red bell pepper, and yellow bell pepper should be sliced into tiny, bite-sized pieces.

Cut the red onion into tiny pieces.

Cut fresh cilantro or parsley into tiny pieces.

Prepare the salad: Combine the cooked quinoa and all of the prepped veggies in a large mixing bowl.

Optional components include: If preferred, top with crumbled feta cheese for a creamy texture and tangy taste.

Include sliced Kalamata olives for a punch of salty flavor.

Make the dressing: Combine the olive oil, balsamic vinegar, minced garlic, Dijon mustard, salt, and pepper in a small mixing bowl.

To taste, adjust the spice.

Dress the salad: Drizzle the dressing over the quinoa and veggie combination.

Mix gently until all of the ingredients are well coated.

Enable flavors to marinate: Cover the salad and refrigerate for at least 30 minutes to enable the flavors to mingle.

This technique enhances the salad's flavor and texture.
Serve and enjoy: Toss the salad one more time before serving.
If preferred, sprinkle with extra herbs or a sprinkling of feta.
Serve chilled, and enjoy the burst of colors and tastes.

Colorful Quinoa Salad Benefits: Quinoa is a complete protein that contains the necessary amino acids. The veggies are abundant in vitamins, minerals, and antioxidants.

Heart-Healthy Fats: The dressing includes monounsaturated fats, which support heart health.

Fiber-rich: Quinoa and veggies are rich in fiber, which assists digestion and promotes a sensation of fullness.

Low in Saturated Fat: The lack of saturated fats makes this salad a heart-healthy option. Versatile and customizable: You may modify the salad to your tastes by adding or deleting elements depending on seasonal availability and personal desire.

Grilled Chicken and Avocado Wraps

Ingredients:

2 skinless, boneless chicken breasts

1 tablespoon of olive oil

1 paprika teaspoon and a half teaspoon cumin

Season with salt and black pepper to taste.

4 spinach or whole-grain wraps

1 avocado (sliced)

1 cup halved cherry tomatoes

1/2 finely chopped red onion

1 cup mixed greens (spinach, arugula, or whatever you prefer)

For sprinkling, use Greek yogurt or your favorite dressing.

To create the marinade:

One lime juice

2 minced garlic cloves

1 tablespoon extra virgin olive oil

1 teaspoon maple syrup or honey

Season with salt and pepper to taste.

Instructions:

Marinate the chicken by adding lime juice, minced garlic, olive oil, honey or maple syrup, salt, and pepper in a mixing bowl.

Place the chicken breasts in the marinade and coat thoroughly. Allow for at least 30 minutes of marinating.

Preheat the grill or grill pan over medium-high heat before cooking the chicken.

Brush the grates with olive oil to prevent them from sticking.

Remove the chicken from the marinade, leaving the excess to drip off, and grill for 6–8 minutes per side, or until fully cooked. The chicken should have a good sear on the exterior and be juicy on the inside.

Allow it to rest for a few minutes before slicing.

Lay out the wraps on a clean surface to prepare them.

Fill each wrap with a hefty handful of mixed greens.

Assemble with Avocado and Tomatoes: On top of the greens, put slices of ripe avocado and split cherry tomatoes.

The avocado's creamy smoothness enhances the tomatoes' burst of freshness.

Sliced Grilled Chicken: Arrange the sliced grilled chicken on top of the greens, avocado, and tomatoes. The scent of the properly roasted chicken adds a delightful element to the ensemble.

Red Onion Sprinkle: Scatter thinly sliced red onions over the mixture. The mild sting of red onion contributes to the overall taste character.

Drizzle with Dressing: Drizzle Greek yogurt or your favorite dressing over the wrap's contents. This offers a creamy, tangy accent that links the tastes together.

Fold and enjoy: Carefully fold the wrap's sides to seal in the scrumptious contents. The wrap is now ready for eating.

Each mouthful delivers a lovely ballet of textures, from the moist softness of the grilled chicken to the creamy richness of the avocado.

Balanced Flavors: The marinade lends a tangy, lemony taste to the chicken, while the avocado adds a buttery richness. The tomatoes create a burst of sweetness, while the red onion provides a bit of spice. This wrap is a nutrient-rich masterpiece, filled with lean protein from the chicken, heart-healthy fats from the avocado, and a spectrum of vitamins and minerals from the veggies.

Versatile Elegance: The adaptability of these wraps is what makes them so attractive. Feel free to experiment with extra ingredients such as cheese, salsa, or your favorite seasonings.

Lentil Soup for Heartwarming Nutrition

Ingredients:

1 cup cleaned and drained dry green or brown lentils

1 big onion, coarsely chopped; 2 carrots, diced 2 celery stalks, chopped 3 garlic cloves, minced 1 can (14 oz) tomato slices 6 cups broth (vegetable or chicken)

1 teaspoon of cumin powder

1 teaspoon of coriander powder

1 tablespoon smoked paprika one bay leaf

2 tablespoons olive oil, seasoned with salt and black pepper to taste

Garnish with fresh parsley or cilantro.

Serve with lemon wedges.

Instructions:

Prepare the lentils.

Rinse and drain the lentils in cold water.

Save these for later use.

Sauté Aromatics: In a large saucepan over medium heat, heat olive oil.

Mix in the chopped onions, carrots, and celery.

Cook until the veggies are cooked and the onions are transparent, approximately 5-7 minutes.

Stir in the minced garlic and the ground spices—cumin, coriander, and smoky paprika.

Continue to simmer for another 1-2 minutes, or until the spices unleash their fragrant essence.

Lentils with Tomatoes: Place the rinsed lentils in the saucepan, followed by the diced tomatoes.

Stir the ingredients together to blend, allowing the lentils to absorb the aromas of the veggies and spices.

Pour in the vegetable or chicken stock, ensuring the lentils are completely immersed.

Add a bay leaf for extra flavor depth. Season to taste with salt and black pepper.

Simmer to Perfection: Bring the soup to a boil, then lower the heat to low.

Cover the pot and simmer the soup for 25–30 minutes, or until the lentils are cooked.

Stir regularly to avoid sticking.

Seasoning: Taste the soup and adjust the seasoning if required. The tastes should be well-balanced, with the lentils and vegetables contributing flavor to the broth.

Ladle the hot lentil soup into bowls and sprinkle with fresh herbs and lemon.

For a burst of herbal freshness, garnish with fresh parsley or cilantro.

Serve each dish with a slice of lemon on the side so that visitors may add a squeeze for a tart finish.

Protein-Rich Lentils: Lentils are a fantastic source of plant-based protein, which is vital for muscle repair and general health. Carrots and celery supply vitamins and minerals, while onions and garlic add a gourmet depth that improves the entire meal.

Balanced Spices: Cumin, coriander, and smoked paprika give not only taste but also important health advantages, including anti-inflammatory effects. Olive oil provides a touch of good fat, which enhances cardiovascular fitness.

Elegance: This lentil soup serves as a diverse canvas. Add greens like spinach or kale, or even a squeeze of fresh lemon for a dramatic explosion of flavor.

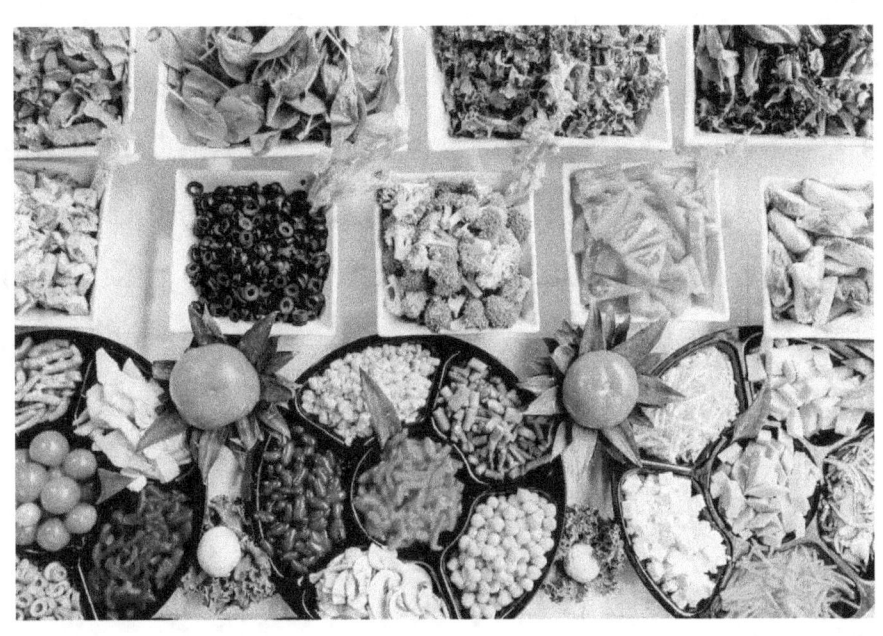

Chapter 4: Dinner Delights for Cardiovascular Wellness

Lemon and Dill Baked Salmon

With this baked salmon recipe, you may experience the delicacies of the sea. Salmon, which is rich in omega-3 fatty acids, takes center stage, seasoned with acidic lemon and pungent dill. Baking maintains the fish's natural moisture, delivering a delicate and heart-healthy protein supply. Serve with steamed asparagus or quinoa for a full evening meal.

Ingredients:
Fillets of salmon Lemon slices, fresh olive oil, and chopped fresh dill To taste, season with salt and pepper.

Quinoa and Vegetable Stir-Fry with a Quinoa and Vegetable Stir-Fry

You may enter the world of plant-powered delight. This colorful salad blends protein-rich quinoa with a variety of crisp veggies to create a heart-healthy and delicious evening option. Stir-frying preserves the nutrients intact while generating a symphony of tastes and textures.

Ingredients: Quinoa has been cooked.
Vegetable stir-fry (bell peppers, broccoli, and snap peas)
Teriyaki sauce or soy sauce
For flavor, add garlic and ginger.
Sesame oil to drizzle

Stuffed Bell Peppers with Turkey and Brown Rice

Stuffed bell peppers are a substantial and healthy alternative for boosting your supper. Lean ground turkey and fiber-rich brown rice give a healthy filling, while colorful bell peppers serve as both a vessel and a delightful garnish. These stuffed peppers are a terrific blend of flavor and heart-consciousness, roasted to perfection.

Ingredients:
Cayenne peppers
Ground turkey that is lean Brown rice, cooked Sauce with tomatoes
Seasonings: onion, garlic, and herbs

Lentil and Sweet Potato

Lentil and sweet potato: Enjoy the warmth of fragrant spices. This plant-based delicacy blends protein-rich lentils with the sweetness of sweet potatoes to produce a heart-healthy supper. The rich scents and brilliant colors of the curry make it a feast for the senses as well as the cardiovascular system.

Ingredients:
Lentils Diced
Sweet potatoes
Coconut cream
Curry ingredients (turmeric, cumin, and coriander)
For flavor, add garlic and ginger. Garnish with fresh cilantro.

Grilled Chicken with Quinoa Salad

Enjoy the simplicity of Grilled Chicken and Quinoa Salad, a supper choice that mixes lean protein with healthy grains and crisp veggies. The grilled chicken offers a savory taste, while the quinoa lends a nutty texture. Drizzle with balsamic vinaigrette for a heart-healthy eating delight.

Ingredients:
Chicken breast
Grilled Quinoa has been cooked.
Greens (arugula and spinach)
Avocado, cherry tomatoes, and cucumber Dressing: balsamic vinaigrette Stew with Eggplant and Chickpeas Eggplant and Chickpea Stew encourages you to enjoy the richness of Mediterranean flavors.
This stew blends the meaty texture of eggplant with the protein-packed flavor of chickpeas to produce a full and heart-healthy dinner. It's a sensation of warmth and well-being, cooked in a tomato-based broth and seasoned with herbs.

Ingredients: eggplant, chickpeas, and cooked tomato sauce.
Flavorings: onion, garlic, and herbs
Toppings: Kalamata olives

Tomato and Basil Whole Grain Pasta

Whole Grain Pasta with Tomato and Basil is a classic with a heart-healthy twist. This fast but filling dish features whole grain pasta for fiber as well as a vivid tomato and basil sauce. Drizzle with olive oil and sprinkle with Parmesan for a meal that pleases both the palette and the heart.

Ingredients:
Pasta made from whole grains
Diced fresh tomatoes
To taste, add fresh basil, minced garlic, olive oil, and red pepper flakes.
Garnish with parmesan cheese.

Skillet with Chickpeas and Spinach

For a fast and healthy supper, turn to the simplicity of a chickpea and spinach skillet. Chickpeas supply plant-based protein, while spinach offers vitamins and minerals. The skillet approach is a simple and heart-healthy solution that does not sacrifice taste.

Ingredients: chickpeas, cleaned and drained spinach leaves, fresh
For taste, add garlic and onion.
Sauce with tomatoes Flavorings: paprika and cumin

Baked Salmon with Lemon-Dill Sauce

Ingredients:

Regarding the salmon: Fillets of salmon Lemon slices, fresh olive oil, and chopped fresh dill

Season with salt and pepper to taste.

To create the lemon-dill sauce: 1/2 cup plain Greek yogurt

1 lemon, zest, and juice

2 tablespoons coarsely chopped fresh dill

1 tbsp. Dijon mustard

Season with salt and pepper to taste.

Instructions:

1. Preparation: Preheat the oven to 375°F (190°C). Line or gently oil a baking dish with parchment paper.

2. Season the fish as follows: Place the salmon fillets in the baking dish that has been prepared. Drizzle olive oil over the fillets, ensuring they are gently covered. Season to taste with salt and pepper. Season the fillets with freshly chopped dill. Place fresh lemon slices on top for a citrus flavor boost.

3. Perfectly Baked: Bake the salmon for 15-20 minutes in a preheated oven, or until the fish flakes easily with a fork. The cooking time will vary depending on the thickness of the fillets.

4. Make the Lemon-Dill Sauce: Combine Greek yogurt, lemon zest, lemon juice, chopped dill, Dijon mustard, salt, and pepper in a mixing bowl. Whisk the ingredients together until fully blended. To taste, adjust the spice.

5. Garnish and serve: Remove the salmon from the oven when it is completely done. Plate the salmon fillets and sprinkle with the lemon-dill sauce. Garnish with more fresh dill for a splash of color.

6. Optional Accompaniments: Serve the baked salmon with steamed asparagus or quinoa for a satisfying and heart-healthy supper.

Salmon that is succulent: The salmon keeps its natural moisture when baked, resulting in a delicate and flaky texture. Salmon, which is abundant in omega-3 fatty acids, enhances heart health and general well-being.

Infusion of Zesty Lemon: Fresh lemon slices, zest, and juice fill the entrée with a fresh citrus fragrance. Lemons contain vitamin C, which is recognized for its antioxidant effects.

Dill Aromatic Embrace: Fresh dill lends a delightful touch to the meal, complementing the salmon's richness. Dill not only increases taste but also offers possible health advantages, including digestive help.

Lemon-Dill Sauce for the Heart: Greek yogurt provides a creamy and healthy basis for the sauce. The lemon and dill bring freshness and depth, while the Dijon mustard provides an acidic zing. The sauce is a low-fat option that combines beautifully with the salmon.

The baked salmon may be served with a number of sides, including steamed vegetables, quinoa, or a light salad, for a diversified eating experience.

Veggie-Packed Stir-Fry with Tofu

Ingredients:

To make the stir-fry:

1 extra-firm tofu block, pressed and cubed vegetables (bell peppers, broccoli, carrots, snap peas)

1 tbsp. sesame seed oil

2 tbsp. soy sauce or tamari

1 teaspoon of hoisin sauce

1 tablespoon of vinegar (rice)

1 tablespoon minced ginger

2 minced garlic cloves

Optional garnish: sesame seeds.

For garnish, chop green onions.

Optional serving suggestions

Instructions for brown rice or quinoa:

1. **Make the tofu:** To remove extra moisture, press the tofu. Cut it up into bite-sized pieces.

2. **Sauté the tofu:** In a wok or big pan, heat the sesame oil over medium-high heat. Heat the tofu cubes until golden brown on both sides, rotating gently. This could take roughly 10 minutes.

3. **Include Aromatics:** Place the tofu on one side of the pan and the minced ginger and garlic on the other. Sauté for 30 seconds, or until aromatic.

4. **Include Vegetables:** Add assorted veggies to the pan. Choose a bright assortment for visual appeal and a diversity of nutrients. Stir-fry the veggies until crisp-tender but still bright.

5. **Construct the sauce:** Combine soy sauce or tamari, hoisin sauce, and rice vinegar on a small plate. Serve the sauce over the tofu and veggies. Toss everything together until fully incorporated.

6. **Decorate and serve:** Garnish the stir-fry with sesame seeds and green onion slices. Serve the veggie-packed Stir-fry over brown rice or quinoa for a substantial and balanced meal.

Veggie-Packed Stir-Fry Harmony: Tofu with Protein

Tofu is the protein powerhouse in this recipe, giving a heart-healthy and delicious plant-based alternative. Vegetables that are crisp and colorful: Bell peppers, broccoli, carrots, and snap peas give a range of colors, textures, and nutrients. **Aromatic Flavors:** Minced ginger and garlic infuse the stir-fry with fragrant flavor, boosting the overall taste profile.

Sweet and savory sauce: The mix of soy sauce, hoisin sauce, and rice vinegar provides a savory and slightly sweet sauce that covers the tofu and veggies.

Cooking with Feeling: Sesame oil offers a nutty taste while keeping the meal heart-healthy. Choosing low-sodium soy sauce or tamari corresponds with heart health even more. Visual appeal garnishes: sesame seeds and chopped green onions give visual appeal as well as extra levels of taste.

Customizable Foundation: Serving the stir-fry over brown rice or quinoa gives a healthy basis that complements the richness of the veggies and tofu.

Quinoa and Black Bean Stuffed Pepper

Ingredients:
To make the stuffed peppers: Bell peppers (various hues)
1 cup of cooked quinoa
1 can of drained and rinsed black beans
1 cup of fresh or frozen corn kernels
1 cup of chopped cherry tomatoes
1/2 cup roughly chopped red onion
1 tablespoon cumin
1 tsp. chili powder
Season with salt and pepper to taste.

1 cup shredded cheese (either cheddar or Mexican mix)
As a garnish: Avocado slices, fresh cilantro, Greek yogurt, or sour cream

Instructions:

1. **Make the peppers:** Preheat the oven to 375 degrees Fahrenheit (190 degrees Celsius). Remove the seeds and membranes from the bell peppers and cut them in half lengthwise.

2. **Prepare Quinoa:** Cook the quinoa according to the package directions. Place aside.

3. **Make the filling:** Combine cooked quinoa, black beans, corn, diced cherry tomatoes, chopped red onion, cumin, chili powder, salt, and pepper in a large mixing bowl. Mix the ingredients until entirely mixed.

4. **Fill the Peppers:** Fill each half of a bell pepper with the quinoa and black bean mixture. Put the filled peppers on a baking dish.

5. **Add the cheese:** Shredded cheese should be put on top of each filled pepper. The cheese will melt and finish golden and bubbling.

6. **Perfectly Baked:** Cover the baking dish with foil and bake for about 25–30 minutes, or until the peppers are cooked.

7. **Decorate and serve:** When the peppers are done, sprinkle with fresh cilantro and serve with avocado slices. For a creamy finish, add a dollop of Greek yogurt or sour cream. Broiling is optional. Broil the filled peppers for a further 2-3 minutes, keeping a careful watch on them to avoid burning, for an additional golden touch on the cheese.

Quinoa and Black Bean Stuffed Peppers Fiesta:Protein-Rich Quinoa

Quinoa is a complete protein that supplies vital amino acids and helps to maintain a balanced and heart-healthy diet. Black beans are rich in fiber. Black beans have a solid texture and are high in fiber, which assists digestion and produces a sensation of fullness.

Vegetable Medley in Various Colors: The combination of cherry tomatoes, red onion, and maize provides a visually pleasing and nutrient-dense vegetable mix.

Spices to impart flavor: Cumin and chili powder give the filling a delicious warmth and depth of flavor. Cheesy Ending: Shredded cheese adds a creamy, savory layer to the meal, producing a gooey, delectable topping.

Freshness garnishes: Each meal is enlivened and refreshed with fresh cilantro, avocado slices, and a dollop of Greek yogurt or sour cream.

Presentation Flexibility: Serve the Quinoa and Black Bean Stuffed Peppers as a main meal or as a wonderful side dish to complement your heart-healthy culinary vacation.

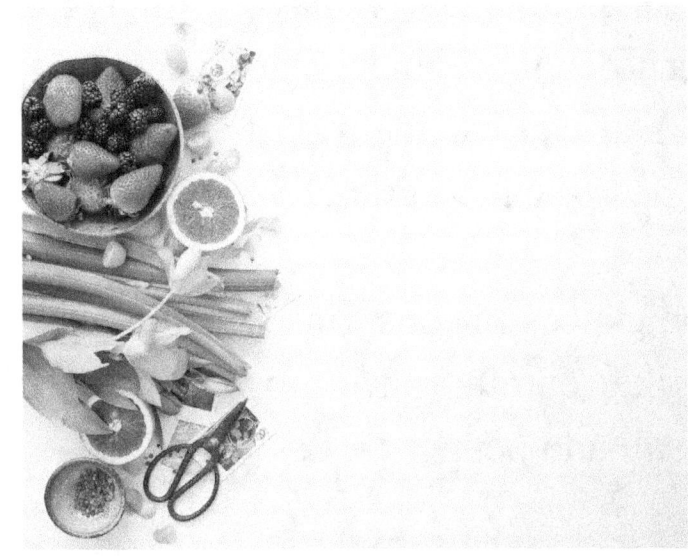

Chapter 5: Snacks for Heart-Smart Munching

Roasted Chickpeas, Crunchy

Crunchy Roasted chickpeas—a snack that blends protein-packed chickpeas with a symphony of spices—transports you to a world of crunch. These small marvels have a great flavor and are an excellent alternative to regular snacks that may be heavy in saturated fats. You can eat them on their own or sprinkle them on salads for a heart-healthy crunch.

Ingredients: chickpeas in cans, rinsed and dried
Olive oil (paprika, cumin, garlic powder, and cayenne pepper) seasoned with salt and pepper

Dark Chocolate Nutty Trail Mix

Nutty Voyage Mix offers a variety of nuts, seeds, and the richness of dark chocolate, bringing you on a journey of heart-healthy delight. This snack is more than just a pleasure for your taste buds; it's also strong in heart-healthy lipids, antioxidants, and energy. Keep a batch on hand for a quick and healthy snack anytime, anywhere.

Ingredients: cashews, walnuts, and almonds
Sunflower and pumpkin seeds Chunks or chips of dark chocolate
Dried fruits (such as apricots and cranberries)

Greek Yogurt and Berries Parfait

Enhance your snacking experience with a Greek yogurt parfait topped with fresh berries. This heart-healthy recipe mixes Greek yogurt's velvety smoothness with the antioxidant-rich sweetness of berries. It's a delicious and nutritious snack that will satisfy your sweet hunger while also improving your health.

Ingredients: Yogurt from Greece Strawberries, blueberries, and raspberries in a mixture Maple or honey syrup Granola for additional crunch

Hummus-Dipped Veggie Sticks

Veggie Sticks and Hummus are a colorful and nutrient-rich snack that accentuates the crispness of fresh vegetables and the creamy charm of hummus. This snack is not only a treat for your taste buds, but it is also a fun way to add crucial vitamins and minerals to your diet.

Ingredients: Sticks of carrot, cucumber, and bell pepper Hummus (bought or homemade)
Cherry tomatoes for an extra flavor boost

Kale Chips Baked Taste

The freshness of Baked Kale Chips, a snack that converts kale leaves into delectable nibbles. These chips, which are high in vitamins and minerals, are a guilt-free alternative to typical potato chips. Season with your choice of seasonings for a unique touch that will delight both your heart and your taste buds.

Ingredients: Kale leaves, fresh Extra virgin olive oil (salt, pepper, nutritional yeast, garlic powder)

Almond Butter Apple Slices

Apple slices with almond butter will fulfill your sweet desire in a heart-healthy way. This snack mixes the natural sweetness of apples with the richness of almond butter, a healthy fat source.

It's a terrific combo that gives a range of flavors as well as health perks.

Ingredients:
Sliced apples (select your favorite sort)
The almond butter
A sprinkle of cinnamon is optional.

Avocado Toast on Whole Wheat Bread

Avocado Toast on Whole Grain Bread is a heart-healthy snack that combines the creamy flavor of avocado with the nutritious richness of whole grains. This snack is a celebration of healthy fats, fiber, and the joy of mindful eating, as well as a treat for your taste buds.

Ingredients: Slices of whole-grain bread Avocado, ripe Juice of a lemon
Seasonings: salt, pepper, and red pepper flakes.

Smoothie with Berries and Chia Seeds

Take a heart-healthy sip with a Berry Smoothie boosted with the nutritious powerhouse of chia seeds. This snack is more than merely a beverage; it's a refreshing surge of antioxidants, vitamins, and omega-3 fatty acids. Blend your favorite berries for a colorful and healthy snack.

Ingredients: Strawberries, blueberries, and raspberries in a mixture Yogurt or almond milk? The seeds of chia For sweetness, use honey or maple syrup.

Roasted Chickpeas with Herbs

Ingredients:
2 cans chickpeas, cleaned and completely dried
2 tbsp. of olive oil
1 tsp. garlic powder
1 tsp. onion powder
1 tsp. dried oregano
1 teaspoon dried thyme

1 tablespoon smoked paprika

1/2 teaspoon cayenne pepper (modify according to taste)

Season with salt and black pepper, to taste.

Garnish with fresh herbs (parsley, cilantro) if preferred.

Instructions:

1. **Preparation and Preheat:** Preheat the oven to 400 degrees Fahrenheit (200 degrees Celsius). Using a clean kitchen towel or paper towel, thoroughly dry the chickpeas. Excess moisture is eliminated to promote optimal crispiness.

2. **Season the chickpeas as follows:** Mix the dry chickpeas with the olive oil, garlic powder, onion powder, dried oregano, dried thyme, smoked paprika, cayenne pepper, salt, and black pepper in a mixing bowl. Toss the chickpeas in the herb-infused spice until completely covered.

3. **Perfectly Roasted:** On a baking sheet lined with parchment paper, distribute the seasoned chickpeas in a single layer. Roast the chickpeas in a preheated oven for 30–40 minutes, or until golden brown and crispy. To ensure uniform roasting, shake the pan or mix the chickpeas halfway through.

4. **Refrigerate and garnish:** Allow to cool slightly before serving the roasted chickpeas. For a splash of herbal freshness, sprinkle with freshly chopped parsley or cilantro.

5. **Keep for Later:** Keep the roasted chickpeas in an airtight jar for up to a week after they have thoroughly cooled. They are best served fresh for optimal crispiness.

Plant-Based Protein: Chickpeas, also known as garbanzo beans, are rich in plant-based protein, making them a tasty and heart-healthy snack. The herb-infused symphony: Garlic powder, onion powder, dried oregano, dried thyme, smoked paprika, and cayenne pepper combine to offer a wonderful mix that turns chickpeas into a savory treat.

Heart-Healthy Olive Oil: The addition of olive oil not only gives a crispy texture but also supplies heart-healthy monounsaturated fats.

Life's Spice: Cayenne pepper provides a touch of heat to foods, not only for flavor but also for its metabolism-boosting effects.

The Magic of Crispy Texture: Drying the chickpeas properly before seasoning is crucial to creating the appropriate crunch. This ensures that the spices adhere correctly, resulting in a lovely exterior.

Freshness garnish: Fresh herbs, such as parsley or cilantro, offer a finishing touch, enhancing the flavor profile.

Snacking Options: Roasted chickpeas may be eaten as a snack on their own, added to salads for crunch, or used as a topping for soups and bowls. The alternatives are simply limited by your imagination.

Nut and Seed Trail Mix

Ingredients:
1 cup raw or gently roasted almonds
1 cup raw or gently roasted walnuts
1/2 cup pepitas (pumpkin seeds)
1/2 cup sunflower seeds
1/2 cup dark chocolate chunks or chips (at least 70% cocoa)
1/2 cup chopped, dried apricots
1/2 cup dried cranberries or cherries, preferably unsweetened
Optional: 1 tablespoon of honey or maple syrup a splash of sea salt

Instructions:
1. **Choose and prepare:** Choose raw or gently toasted almonds and walnuts for a stunning textural contrast. If the pumpkin and sunflower seeds are raw, gently roast them for a few minutes in a dry skillet over medium heat until aromatic. Allow for cooling.

2. **Make the base:** Combine the almonds, walnuts, pumpkin seeds, and sunflower seeds in a large mixing dish.

3. **Include the indulgences:** Incorporate extravagance into the dish by adding dark chocolate chunks or chips. Use dried apricots and cranberries to enhance sweetness and chewiness.

4. **Add a Bonus (Optional):** If you wish to add additional sweetness, sprinkle honey or maple syrup over the mixture. To coat evenly, stir the mixture.

5. **Add a pinch of sea salt:** A sprinkling of sea salt intensifies the taste and gives a savory balance to the sweetness.

6. **Combine and store:** Gently mix all of the ingredients until thoroughly incorporated. For on-the-go pleasure, put the Nut and Seed Trail Mix in an airtight container or divide it into snack-sized bags.

7. **Energize Your Adventures:** Let the Nut & Seed Trail Mix be your partner for a healthy and active break, whether you're hitting the trails, working at your desk, or enjoying a moment of leisure.

Almonds and Walnuts

Almonds and walnuts are abundant in nutrients. Almonds and walnuts are rich in monounsaturated fats, omega-3 fatty acids, and other critical elements. Protein-Rich Seeds: Pumpkin seeds and sunflower seeds give a delightful crunch while also supplying plant-based protein, fiber, and a range of vitamins and minerals.

Dark Chocolate Delectable

Dark chocolate chunks not only satisfy your sweet craving but also deliver antioxidants and may boost heart health.

Dried Fruits with Chew

indulgence that not only fulfills your chocolate cravings but also celebrates the heart-healthy richness of avocados. This mousse is a smooth symphony of flavors that mixes rich dark chocolate with creamy avocados to produce a guilt-free treat that will please both your taste buds and your well-being.

Ingredients: avocados that have matured 70% cacao or higher dark chocolate
Cocoa powder without sugar
Honey/maple syrup
Vanilla flavoring with a splash of sea salt
Garnish with fresh berries.

Berry Chia Seed Pudding

Berry Chia Seed Pudding is a jar of antioxidant-rich bliss that blends the health benefits of chia seeds with the vibrant sweetness of berries. This pudding is a delectable treat that not only meets your sweet craving but also gives a healthy dosage of omega-3 fatty acids and fiber, resulting in heart-healthy pleasure.

Ingredients: The seeds of chia Yogurt from Greece Milk made from almonds
Strawberries, blueberries, and raspberries in a combination
Honey/maple syrup
Sliced almonds for garnish

Vanilla Extract Almond Flour Banana Bread

Banana bread is a traditional treat recreated with nutrient-rich almond flour and juicy bananas. This heart-friendly recipe keeps the moist and delicate features of classic banana bread while adding healthy fats, protein, and the natural sweetness of bananas.

Ingredients:
Almond meal
Bananas that have matured
Eggs
Yogurt from Greece

The oil of coconut
The maple syrup
Vanilla flavoring
Baking powder
Cinnamon (optional)
Chopped walnuts

Heartwarming Oatmeal Raisin Cookies

Enjoy the warmth of Oatmeal Raisin Cookies with a healthy twist—a cookie jar staple that mixes the nutritional richness of oats with the natural sweetness of raisins. These cookies are a wonderful treat packed with fiber, antioxidants, and a calming taste that conjures up the delight of handmade sweets.

Ingredients:
Whole-grain flour
The oil of coconut Honey/maple syrup
Eggs

Vanilla flavoring
Cinnamon
Baking powder Raisins

Fruits and Vegetables Sorbet

A Vibrant and Cool Citrus Refreshment Fresh Fruit Sorbet is a tasty and gorgeous dessert that captures the pleasure of summer in every mouthful. This sorbet celebrates natural sweetness from a combination of fresh fruits, delivering a guilt-free choice that tantalizes your taste buds while also providing a boost of vitamins and hydration.

Ingredients:
Fresh fruits (strawberries, mango, kiwi, and pineapple) assorted
Orange, lime, or lemon juice, freshly squeezed
Optional: maple syrup or honey garnished with mint leaves

Wholesome Carrot Cake Bites

Wholesome Carrot Cake Bites are a bite-sized treat that captures the flavor of carrot cake in a heart-conscious shape. These small morsels are packed with shredded carrots, almonds, and warming spices, delivering a wonderful blend of sweetness and nutty crunch without the guilt.

Ingredients:
Carrots, shredded almond meal
Pecans or walnuts
Dates
The oil of coconut
Nutmeg
Cinnamon
Vanilla flavoring Coating: unsweetened shredded coconut

Grilled Pineapple with Honey and Mint

Grilled Pineapple with Honey and Mint is a tropical-inspired dish that turns fresh pineapple into a caramelized delight. The innate sweetness of pineapple is amplified by grilling, and a drizzle of honey and a sprinkle of mint elevate this simple delicacy to a refreshing conclusion that fulfills your sweet desires with refinement.

Ingredients:
Slices of fresh pineapple
Honey
Garnish with fresh mint leaves.

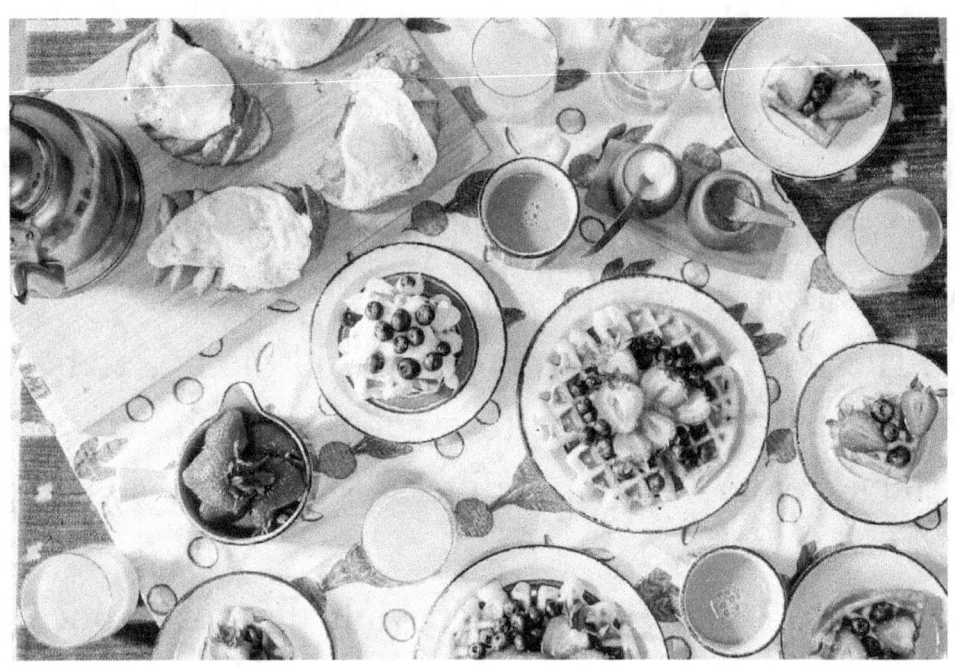

Dark Chocolate and Berry Clusters

Ingredients:
1 cup chopped dark chocolate (70% cocoa or more)
1 cup berries (strawberries, blueberries, and raspberries)
1 tablespoon of coconut oil
1/2 cup chopped nuts (almonds, walnuts, or a combination)
Optional: 1 tablespoon of honey or maple syrup a splash of sea salt
To line the tray, use parchment paper.

Instructions:

1. First, melt the dark chocolate. Melt the dark chocolate in a heatproof dish over a double boiler or in short bursts in the microwave. Stir until totally smooth.

2. **Make the fruit and nut mixture:** Add the mixed berries and chopped nuts of your choice to a separate dish. This generates the cluster's center, which delivers a rush of sweetness and crunch.

3. **Incorporate Dark Chocolate:** Melt the dark chocolate and sprinkle it over the fruit and nut mixture. Incorporate the ingredients gradually until the berries and almonds are equally covered in chocolate.

4. Stir in the coconut oil and sweetener (optional). If desired, blend the mixture with coconut oil, honey, or maple syrup. This increases the chocolate's smoothness and gives it a touch of sweetness. Add a teaspoon of sea salt to the mixture for a fantastic balance of tastes.

5. **Make Clusters:** Spoon tiny bits of the mixture into clusters on a tray equipped with parchment paper. Make sure they are equally spaced to enable easy removal once set.

6. **Place in the refrigerator to set:** Refrigerate the dish for at least 30 minutes to enable the clusters to harden. This also assists in the hardening of the chocolate.

7. **Plate and enjoy:** Remove the clusters from the refrigerator when they have firmed up. Remove the clusters from the parchment paper and serve immediately.

Dark Chocolate Delectable

Dark chocolate with a cocoa level of 70% or higher not only satisfies your sweet taste but also delivers a multitude of antioxidants and possible heart health advantages.

Medley of Mixed Berries

Strawberries, blueberries, and raspberries combine to offer natural sweetness, fiber, and a range of vitamins to the clusters.

Crunchy Nut Combination

Almonds, walnuts, or a combination of nuts deliver a delicious crunch and heart-healthy lipids in each mouthful. Coconut oil is healthy for your heart. Coconut oil provides smoothness to the chocolate while also delivering heart-healthy lipids.

Optional Sweetener:

Honey or Maple Syrup

The addition of honey or maple syrup is optional, enabling you to customize the sweetness of the clusters to your liking.

1 teaspoon sea salt: Sea salt gives a salty contrast to the entire taste profile, complementing the sweetness.

Clusters that are ideally positioned: The shape of the clusters enables portion control while also providing a pleasant and luxurious experience.

Indulgence in Antioxidant-Rich Foods: Berries and dark chocolate are both abundant in antioxidants, making these clusters a tasty treat that enhances overall health.

Heart-Healthy Banana Bread

Ingredients:

Mashed 2 to 3 ripe bananas; a third of a cup of Greek yogurt

1/4 cup melted coconut oil

1/4 cup applesauce, unsweetened

1/2 cup maple syrup or honey

2 large eggs a teaspoon vanilla extract

1 cup whole wheat flour

1 tsp. baking soda a half teaspoon of cinnamon

1/2 cup chopped walnuts or pecans (optional)

1/4 teaspoon salt

Instructions:

1. Preheat and get ready. Preheat the oven to 350 degrees Fahrenheit (175 degrees Celsius). Set aside a standard-sized loaf pan that has been greased.

2. **Mashed Bananas:** Mash the ripe bananas with a fork or potato masher in a large mixing bowl until smooth.

3. **Combine Wet Ingredients:** To the mashed bananas, add Greek yogurt, melted coconut oil, applesauce, honey or maple syrup, eggs, and vanilla extract. Blend until thoroughly combined.

4. **Mix together the dry ingredients:** Combine whole wheat flour, baking soda, cinnamon, and salt in a separate bowl.

5. **Combine dry and wet ingredients:** Add the dry ingredients to the liquid ones gradually, stirring until just combined. Take care not to overmix.

6. **Optional nut toppings:** To add a delicious crunch to your banana bread batter, mix in chopped walnuts or pecans, if preferred.

7. **Pour into the pan:** Spread the batter evenly into the prepared loaf pan.

8. **Perfectly Baked:** Bake for 50–60 minutes, or until a toothpick inserted into the center comes out clean or with a few damp crumbs.

9. **Allow to cool before slicing:** Allow the banana bread to rest for 10–15 minutes in the pan before transferring it to a wire rack to cool completely before slicing.

10. **Serve and Have Fun:** Enjoy each heart-healthy piece of this scrumptious banana bread. It may be eaten on its own, toasted, or with a tiny spread of almond butter for a heart-healthy twist.

Ripe bananas provide natural sweetness as well as potassium, vitamins, and dietary fiber.

Moisture in Greek Yogurt

Greek yogurt adds creaminess and wetness to banana bread while also providing protein and probiotics.

Coconut oil contains heart-healthy fats: Melted coconut oil adds heart-healthy saturated fats to the dish, making it moist and supple.

Sweeteners from nature: Sweetening the banana bread with honey or maple syrup eliminates the need for refined sugars, making it a heart-healthy option.

Nutrients in Whole Wheat Flour: Whole wheat flour replaces refined flour in bread, adding fiber, vitamins, and minerals.

Cinnamon's warmth: Cinnamon not only provides a pleasant warmth, but it also has potential health benefits, including anti-inflammatory properties.

Nut Crunch (Optional): If used, chopped walnuts or pecans provide heart-healthy fats and a lovely crunch to each slice.

Diverse Pleasure: Heart-Healthy Banana Bread is flexible, serving as a breakfast treat, a filling snack, or a guilt-free dessert.

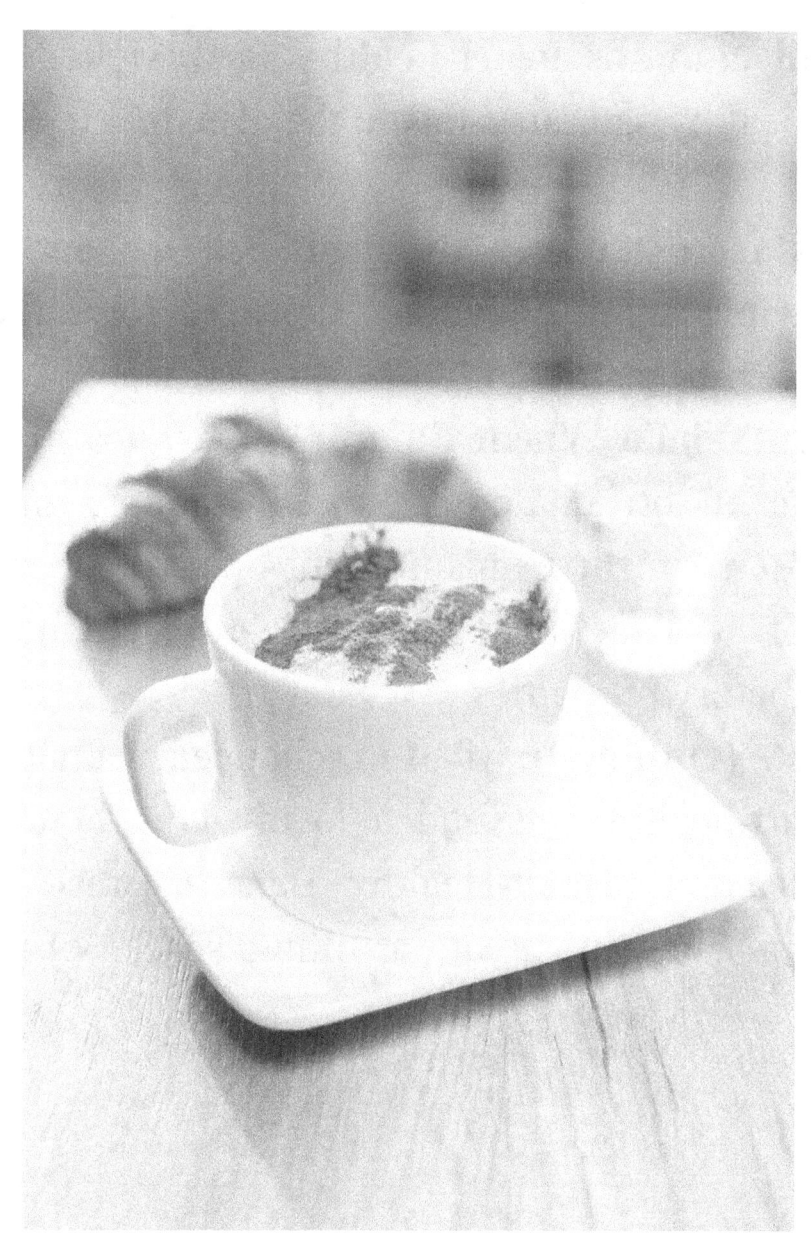

Berry Bliss Smoothie Popsicles

Ingredients:

1 cup hulled and halved strawberries a half-cup of blueberries

1/2 cup of fresh raspberries

1 cup of plain Greek yogurt

2 tbsp. honey or maple syrup a teaspoon vanilla extract

1/4 cup almond milk (or your chosen milk)

Popsicle Sticks and Molds

Instructions:

1. **Magic Berry Medley:** Strawberries, blueberries, raspberries, Greek yogurt, honey or maple syrup, vanilla extract, and almond milk in a blender.

2. **Blend until smooth:** Blend the ingredients until smooth and entirely incorporated. The finished result should be a colorful, berry-infused smoothie foundation.

3. **Prepare popsicle molds:** Fill popsicle molds halfway with the berry smoothie mixture, leaving a little room at the top for expansion after freezing.

4. **Insert the sticks:** Insert popsicle sticks into the middle of each mold, ensuring they are straight.

5. **Perfectly Freeze:** Place the filled popsicle molds in the freezer for at least 4-6 hours, or until totally firm.

6. **Remove the mold and enjoy:** When the Berry Bliss Smoothie Popsicles have frozen firm, remove them from the molds by briefly running the bottom under warm water. This loosens the popsicles and enables simple removal.

7. **Enjoy the bliss:** Berry Delight Smoothie Popsicles bring frozen joy. Each mouthful is a burst of seasonal delight, whether enjoyed on a hot summer day or as a healthful dessert.

The Berry Bliss Smoothie Popsicles Symphony

Strawberries, blueberries, and raspberries combine to create a range of tastes, colors, and antioxidants, evoking the spirit of summer.

Elegance in Creamy Yogurt: Greek yogurt lends a creamy, rich texture to the popsicles while also delivering protein and probiotics for a healthy treat.

Nature's Sweetness Amplified: Honey or maple syrup provides sweetness while boosting the natural sugars inherent in ripe berries.

A Smidgeon of Vanilla Magic: Vanilla essence gives a delicate depth of flavor to the popsicles, enriching the whole tasting experience.

Smoothness of Almond Milk: Almond milk, or any milk of choice, lends a nutty smoothness to the recipe, ensuring that the popsicles freeze to a beautiful texture.

Artistry with Popsicle Molds: The popsicle molds serve as a canvas for you to create vivid, artistic frozen joys that are as visually beautiful as they are delectable.

Summer Portable Joy: Berry Bliss Smoothie Popsicles are a portable treat that transmits the joy of summer wherever you go.

Chapter 6: Beverages That Love Your Heart

Hibiscus Berry Iced Tea

This red elixir mixes the floral tones of hibiscus with the aroma of berries to produce a scrumptious drink that not only tantalizes your taste buds but also benefits your heart health with each sip.

Ingredients:
Tea bags with hibiscus Strawberries, blueberries, and raspberries in a combination of mint leaves, fresh
Optional: honey or agave syrup.

Cubes of Ice Citrus-Infused Water

Enhance your hydration experience with Citrus Infused Water, a delicious composition that mixes the freshness of citrus fruits with the clarity of water. This tasty beverage not only keeps you hydrated but also fills your day with the stimulating fragrance of citrus, which is recognized for its heart-healthy characteristics.

Ingredients:
Lemon wedges, wedges of lime
Sliced oranges
Mint leaves, fresh
Cubes of ice

Green Tea with Lemon and Ginger

This is a beverage that blends green tea's antioxidant properties with the zing of citrus and the warmth of ginger. This heart-warming infusion is a sip of calm that enhances general well-being.

Ingredients:
Bags of green tea
Lemon wedges

Honey or maple syrup (optional), thinly sliced fresh ginger

Berry-Beet Smoothie

A beverage that mixes the sweetness of berries with the earthy depth of beets. This smoothie is not only tasty; it's also a heart-healthy elixir filled with antioxidants and critical minerals.

Ingredients: Berries (strawberries, blueberries, raspberries)
Greek yogurt cooked and peeled beets
Agave or honey syrup
Milk made from almonds
Cubes of ice

Minty Cucumber Cooler

This is a delightful drink that mixes the sharpness of cucumber with the stimulating touch of mint. This hydrating drink not only quenches thirst but also enhances heart health thanks to its hydrating and refreshing characteristics.

Ingredients:
Slices of cucumber, mint leaves, and fresh lemon wedges
Optional: honey or agave syrup.
Cubes of ice

Golden Turmeric Latte

This is a beverage that blends turmeric's anti-inflammatory properties with the smoothness of milk. This golden elixir is a calming treat that not only excites your senses but also helps your overall health.

Ingredients:
Powdered turmeric
Dairy or plant-based milk
Cinnamon

Powdered ginger
Optional: honey or maple syrup.

Pomegranate Green Tea Smoothie

This smoothie is not only tasty, but it is also an energy drink that supports heart health.

Ingredients:
Seeds of pomegranate brewed and cooled green tea
Banana
Spinach stems
Yogurt from Greece
Agave or honey syrup
Cubes of ice

Refreshing Green Tea Lemonade

Ingredients:
2 sachets of green tea
2 cups of boiling water
1/4 cup honey or agave syrup (to taste)
1/2 cup freshly squeezed lemon juice (approximately 3–4 lemons)
Cubes of ice
Optional garnishes: lemon slices and mint leaves

Instructions:
1. Start by brewing the green tea. Let the green tea bags steep in boiling water for 3-5 minutes to enable the flavors to infuse. Remove the tea bags and leave them aside to cool to room temperature.
2. **Adjust the sweetness to taste:** Adjust the sweetness of the brewed green tea with honey or agave syrup to suit. Stir well to obtain equitable dispersion.

3. **Squeeze in some fresh lemon juice:** Juice the lemons to create roughly 1/2 cup of fresh lemon juice. Adjust the amount to your optimum degree of tartness.

4. **Mix together green tea and lemon juice:** Combine the brewed green tea and fresh lemon juice in a pitcher. To combine the flavors, gently whisk them together.

5. Allow the mixture to cool. Refrigerate the pitcher to cool the green tea lemonade. This enables the tastes to blend and increases the overall refreshing experience.

6. **Serve with ice:** Pour the green tea lemonade over ice cubes in separate glasses when it has cooled. The ice offers a refreshing and revitalizing touch.

7. **Optional garnish for visual appeal:** Garnish each glass with a slice of lemon and a sprig of fresh mint on the rim. This approach not only increases the visual appeal but also adds a slight smell.

8. **Sip and Relax:** Take a time to appreciate the delightful mix of green tea and lemon after you've brewed and garnished your green tea lemonade. Allow the energetic flavors to both relax and refresh your senses.

Lemonade Green Tea

This is recognized for its strong antioxidant content, which may aid with heart health and general well-being.

Lemon Citrus Zing: Freshly squeezed lemon juice not only gives a zesty taste to the drink, but it also delivers vitamin C and a wonderful brightness.

Natural Sweetener (Honey or Agave): Honey or agave syrup gives natural sweetness, improving flavor without the use of refined sugars. Crispiness from the ice: Adding ice cubes to the green tea lemonade adds a layer of crispness, making each drink cold and vibrant.

Garnishes for Visual Delight: Optional garnishes of lemon slices and mint leaves not only add visual appeal but also a slight smell to the drink. Sweetness may be customized: The sweetness level is adjustable, enabling you to adapt the green tea lemonade to your liking.

Perfect Hydration Partner: Refreshing Green Tea Lemonade is the ideal partner for keeping hydrated with elegance, whether enjoyed on a hot day or as a peaceful evening drink.

Antioxidant-Packed Berry Smoothie

Ingredients:
1 cup berries (strawberries, blueberries, and raspberries)
1/2 cup of fresh blackberries
1/2 cup plain Greek yogurt
1 tbsp. chia seeds
1 tbsp. honey (or agave syrup)
1 cup almond milk (or your chosen milk)
Ice cubes are optional.

Instructions:
1. **Magic Berry Medley:** Blend the mixed berries, blackberries, Greek yogurt, chia seeds, honey or agave syrup, and almond milk in a blender.
2. **Blend until silky smooth:** Blend the ingredients until they are silky smooth. The rich colors of the berries should combine to form a delectable blend.
3. **Verify Consistency:** If the smoothie is too thick, add additional almond milk and combine until the appropriate consistency is obtained.

4. **Optionally, add ice cubes:** Add a handful of ice cubes to the blender and swirl until the smoothie reaches your preferred temperature.

5. **Ladle into a glass:** Pour the antioxidant-rich berry smoothie into a tall glass, savoring the bright colors.

6. **Optional garnish for visual delight:** Garnish the smoothie with a few whole berries for a distinctive touch. This not only contributes to the visual beauty, but it also gives a blast of freshness with each sip.

7. **Drink and Bask in Radiance:** Take a minute to taste the berry-packed sweetness with your glass in hand. Each sip should be a celebration of the antioxidants that increase your health.

Hydrating Infused Water Combos

Explore a world of hydration that goes beyond the usual with Hydrating Infused Water Combos, a selection of exquisite combinations that convert basic water into a symphony of tastes. These infused water combinations not only increase your hydration but also deliver a blast of natural taste without the need for added sweets or artificial chemicals. May you learn the talent of keeping hydrated with a touch of culinary flair.

1. **Cucumber Mint Splash:** A Refreshing Cooler Ingredients: cucumber, cut Fresh mint leaves, ice cubes, and water In a pitcher, add cucumber slices and fresh mint leaves. Fill the pitcher halfway with water and ice cubes. enable it to rest for at least 30 minutes to enable the flavors to mingle. Pour over ice and enjoy the cold, refreshing delight.

2. **Citrus Berry Burst:** A Tangy Sweet Symphony Ingredients: lemon slices, sliced Ice cubes with fresh berries (strawberries, blueberries, raspberries) Instructions for Using Water: Combine sliced lemon, sliced lime, and fresh berries in a pitcher. Fill the

pitcher halfway with water and ice cubes. Allow at least 1 hour to infuse to bring out the citrus and berry tastes. Pour over ice for a refreshing rush of zesty sweetness.

3. **Pineapple Basil Bliss:** Tropical Calm in Every Sip

Ingredients:

Pineapple slices, fresh basil leaves, and fresh cubes of ice

Instructions for Using Water:

In a pitcher, add fresh pineapple slices and basil leaves.
Fill the pitcher halfway with water and ice cubes.
Allow at least 2 hours for the tropical flavor to emerge.
Pour over ice for a pleasant taste of pineapple and basil.

Watermelon Rose Refresher

Ingredients:
Watermelon cubes
Fresh rose petals (pesticide-free and tasty)
Cubes of ice

Instructions for Using Water:

In a pitcher, add cubed watermelon and fresh rose petals.

Fill the pitcher halfway with water and ice cubes.

Allow it to marinate for at least 1 hour to achieve a subtle floral sweetness.

Pour over ice for a delightful watermelon rose cocktail.

Ginger Lemon Zest

A Zingy Awakening Ingredients: ginger, sliced lemon segments Cubes of ice Instructions for Using Water: In a pitcher, mix the sliced ginger and lemon. Fill the pitcher halfway with water and ice cubes. Allow at least 30 minutes for the zingy spices to enter the water. Pour over ice for a rejuvenating ginger lemon zest drink.

Tranquil Berry Delight with Berry-Lavender Infusion Ingredients: strawberries, blueberries, and raspberries in a combination Ice cubes with fresh lavender sprigs Instructions for Using Water: In a pitcher, blend mixed berries and fresh lavender sprigs. Fill the pitcher halfway with water and ice cubes. Allow it to soak for at least 2 hours to absorb the relaxing scent of lavender. For a berry-lavender infusion, serve over ice.

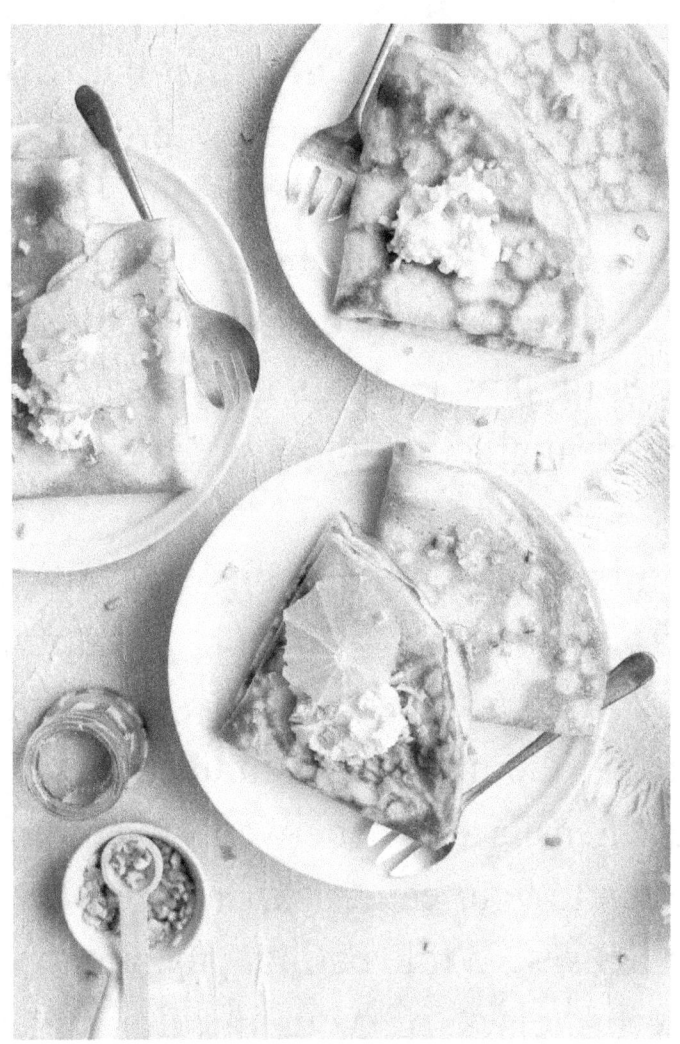

Chapter 7: Mindful Eating Habits for Heart Health

Mindful eating is a timeless practice that helps you relish every mouthful in a world that often hurries through meals. Slowing down the speed of your meals not only increases the enjoyment of eating but also provides your body with the time it needs to indicate fullness, decreasing overeating. In this part, we'll look at the advantages of slow eating and present practical ways for adopting this mindful practice into your everyday life.

Important Points: Take smaller bits and concentrate on the textures, tastes, and scents of each mouthful. Chew with intention: Chew your meal completely, enabling the digestive process to begin in the mouth and indicating satisfaction to the brain. Put your utensils down between meals to create pauses that draw attention to your eating experience.

Activate Your Senses: While eating, pay attention to the colors, scents, and even noises of your meal, immersing yourself entirely in the process of nutrition.

Portion Control: Achieving a balance of quantity and quality portion awareness is an essential part of mindful eating, highlighting the requirement of balancing the amount and quality of food ingested. This describes strategies for assessing portion sizes instinctively, enabling you to retain a good relationship with food while simultaneously supporting your heart health objectives.

Important Points: Use smaller dishes to visually provide a proper portion, producing an impression of fullness without excess.

Pay Attention to Hunger Cues: Pay attention to your body's hunger and fullness signals and allow them to dictate your portion amounts.

Balanced Plate: Aim for a nutrient-dense dish that contains lean meats, complete grains, and colorful fruits and veggies. Distractions should be avoided. To be alert to your body's cues, minimize distractions such as television or technological gadgets during meals.

Accepting Nutrient-Dense Options

Fueling your heart nutrient-dense meals are the cornerstone of mindful eating for cardiovascular health. This goes into the bright world of comprehensive, nutrient-dense meals that include necessary vitamins, minerals, and antioxidants to boost heart health. Learn how to cook meals that not only taste wonderful but also contribute to your body's health and energy.

Important Points:
Colorful Variety: Include a rainbow of fruits and vegetables in your diet to gain a wide variety of nutrients.

Lean Proteins: Choose lean protein sources such as fish, chicken, beans, and lentils to improve heart-healthy lipids and amino acids.

Whole Grains: For fiber, B vitamins, and long-lasting energy, pick whole grains such as quinoa, brown rice, and oats.

Healthy Fats: To promote cardiovascular health, eat sources of healthy fats such as avocados, almonds, and olive oil.

Mindful Hydration

Water nutrition for your body hydration is vital for heart health, and attentive drinking goes beyond simple intake. In this part, you'll learn about the significance of keeping hydrated and the thoughtful behaviors that may help you improve your connection with water while also enhancing your general well-being.

Important Points: Drink water thoughtfully, appreciating each sip and enabling your body to absorb fluids effectively. **Incorporate herbal teas:** Herbal teas are a pleasant and calming alternative that is caffeine-free and strong in antioxidants. **Infused Water Rituals:** Make infused water combinations that not only hydrate but also infuse natural tastes into your beverages.

Mindful Eating and Gratitude

Developing a Healthy Relationship with Food Gratitude—a sincere appreciation for the sustenance food provides—is at the center of mindful eating for heart health. This part digs into the practice of mindful appreciation, creating a good connection with food, and reinforcing the concept that each meal is a chance to care for your body and spirit.

Important Points: Take a minute before your supper to express thanks for the food on your plate and the hands that prepared it. Consider the sources of your food, respecting the work of farmers, producers, and everyone else involved in getting it to your table.

Mindful Preparation: Make a concerted effort to prepare your meals, infusing the process with significance and thanks.

Portion Control and Balance

A lighthouse for healthy eating habits portion management and balance emerge as guiding principles in the complex fabric of mindful eating, bringing us toward a happy relationship with food. This goes into the skill of recognizing and appreciating portion management, the necessity of balancing nutrients, and how these disciplines work together to enhance general health and well-being.

The Visual Guide to Understanding Portion Control

Portion management starts with a visual awareness of serving sizes. Familiarize yourself with essential measures so that you can estimate suitable quantities for diverse food types. Pay attention to your body. Pay attention to hunger and fullness signals. Before going for seconds, think about whether you truly need additional food. Listening to your body is an essential element of portion control.

Mindful Eating Techniques: Engage in mindful eating by enjoying each mouthful. Slowly eating and enjoying the flavors offers your body the time it needs to sense fullness, minimizing overeating.

Smaller plates, better decisions: Choose smaller plates to give the appearance of a bigger plate. This psychological method assists in portion control and pleasure increase.

Nutritional Balance Techniques: The Plate Technique: Accept the plate strategy, which entails splitting your plate into portions for various food groups. Set aside half for vegetables, a quarter for lean proteins, and the final quarter for whole grains. Include colorful variety: A balanced plate is one that is colorful. Include a variety of fruits and vegetables in a variety of colors to supply a wide range of nutrients.

Lean Proteins for Long-Term Energy: Choose lean proteins like chicken, fish, tofu, and lentils. These not only supply vital amino acids but also add to a sensation of fullness.

Whole Grains for Fiber and Nutrition: Select whole grains, such as quinoa, brown rice, and oats. These grains provide fiber, vitamins, and long-lasting energy, all of which contribute to a well-rounded and balanced diet.

Moderate Consumption of Healthy Fats: Avocados, almonds, and olive oil are all fantastic sources of healthy fats. These fats boost heart health and add taste to your meals.

Conscious Hydration: Drinks play a significant part in equilibrium. Choose water as your main beverage and reduce sugary beverages. Staying hydrated is a key factor in overall wellness.

Practical Implementation Advice: Snacks should be pre-portioned. To minimize mindless chewing, break food into different parts. This basic method encourages conscious eating and assists with calorie control.

Use Measuring Instruments: When cooking meals, use measuring cups, spoons, or a food scale. This assures accuracy and helps teach your eyes to distinguish acceptable proportions.

Be Aware of Outside Influences: Be conscious of external circumstances that may alter portion sizes, such as huge restaurant meals. To retain balance, try sharing a meal or bringing leftovers home.

Maintain a Food Journal: Keep a food journal to document your meals and portion amounts. This exercise develops self-awareness and gives insights into your eating practices. Enjoy treats mindfully. Indulge in treats occasionally, but do it intelligently. Savor the tastes and be cautious of portion amounts to establish a balance between pleasure and moderation.

Smart Substitutions for Heart-Healthy Cooking

1. **Whole Grains vs. Refined:** The replacement of whole grains for refined grains is a cornerstone of heart-healthy cuisine. Whole grains like quinoa, brown rice, and oats contain additional fiber, vitamins, and minerals, which aid with cardiovascular health.

Brown Rice: For a heartier, fiber-rich option, substitute white rice with brown rice.

Quinoa: Quinoa is a flexible and protein-rich alternative to refined grains.

Whole Wheat Flour: For baking and cooking, use whole wheat flour instead of refined flour.

2. **Heart-Healthy Fats:** Choosing the appropriate lipids is vital for heart health. Replace saturated fats with heart-healthy alternatives such as olive oil, avocado oil, and nut oils. These

options contain monounsaturated fats, which boost cardiovascular health.

Olive oil may be used in place of butter or lard in cooking and salad dressings.

Avocado Oil: Avocado oil offers a delicate, nutty taste to high-heat cooking. Drizzle almond or walnut oil over foods as a finishing touch for a heart-healthy taste boost.

3. **Lean Proteins:** lean proteins is an essential element of heart-healthy cuisine. As an alternative to red and processed meats, pick chicken, fish, beans, and legumes. These solutions provide needed nutrients while eliminating saturated fat.

Chicken or Turkey: For a decreased protein source, swap chicken or turkey for red meat in recipes. Fatty fish, such as salmon, mackerel, or trout, are rich in omega-3 fatty acids and may aid your heart.

Plant-Based Proteins: For heart-healthy choices, check into plant-based protein sources such as lentils, beans, and tofu.

4. **Herbs & Spices:** Boosting flavor without adding sodium reduced salt consumption is crucial for heart health. Instead of using too much salt, utilize herbs and spices to improve the flavor of your dish. This not only adds depth to tastes, but it also possesses antioxidants and anti-inflammatory effects.

Fresh Herbs: For a bright, sodium-free taste, use fresh herbs such as basil, cilantro, and parsley.

Spice blends: Make your own spice blends using cumin, coriander, turmeric, and other heart-healthy spices.

Citrus Zest: Grate citrus zest for a flavor boost without adding salt.

5 **Natural Sweeteners:** Reducing additional sugars is vital for heart-healthy cooking. To add sweetness to your foods, use natural sweeteners such as honey, maple syrup, or agave nectar instead of manufactured sugars.

Honey or Maple Syrup: To add sweetness to recipes, replace honey or maple syrup with refined sugar.

Agave Nectar: Agave nectar may be used as an alternative sweetener, notably in drinks and sweets.

Fruit Purees: Use fruit purees, such as applesauce, in baking to offer natural sweetness.

6. **Plant-Based Milk:** Dairy alternatives for better heart health plant-based milk solutions provide heart-healthy choices for individuals seeking dairy alternatives. Almond milk, soy milk, and oat milk are all abundant in nutrients and may be readily blended into a number of dishes.

Almond Milk: Replace dairy milk in cereals, smoothies, and baking with almond milk.

Soy Milk: As a dairy-free replacement, use soy milk in savory and sweet meals.

Oat Milk: Use oat milk in coffee or as a basis for rich recipes to experience its velvety texture.

Eating with Awareness and Gratitude

Eating with Awareness and Gratitude: A heart and soul feast meals in today's fast-paced society are often short interludes, a means to an end rather than a holy act of feeding. However, the capacity to eat with attention and appreciation urges us to convert these events into a feast for the heart and spirit. This exercise goes beyond routine eating; it is a voyage of attention, a celebration of tastes, and a recognition of the abundance that adorns our tables.

The mindful presence Ritual: Inhale, exhale, and savor: Begin each meal with a few minutes of deep breathing. Allow the scent of your meal to delight your senses as you inhale deeply and gradually exhale. This one movement makes a connection between the outside world and the nourishment in front of you. **Activate Your Senses:** Engage all of your senses as you sit down to eat. Examine the colors, textures, and presentation of your food. Inhale the smells that drift through the air. Allow your eyes to feast on your meal's visual poetry. Slow down and appreciate more. Resist the impulse to speed through your meal. Each swallow is a chance to appreciate the symphony of flavors. Chew carefully, allowing the flavors to develop on your palette. Allow eating to become a mindful experience, a meditation in action.

Before You Take Your First Bite: Give thanks for a minute before your first mouthful. Recognize the hands who made the dinner, the food that traveled to your table, and the circumstances that led to this wonderful confluence of time and nutrition.

Keeping a Gratitude Journal: Consider creating a gratitude notebook for your culinary experiences. Make a note of the tastes you prefer, the sensations that tickled your taste buds, and the moments of connection shared around the table.

Consider Abundance: Consider the gems before you during your lunch break. Recognize the richness in the diversity of colors, tastes, and nutrients that contribute to your well-being, whether it's a simple home-cooked supper or an extravagant spread. **Portions Awareness:** Be aware of portion sizes and appreciate each meal without the impulse to eat more than is required. This technique not only builds appreciation for the nutrients offered, but it also creates a healthy connection with food.

Zone Devoid of Technology: Make mealtime a technology-free zone. Turn off devices, turn off alarms, and make dining a conscious effort. This devoted time helps you to connect with your food, your company, and the present situation.

Thank You Notes: If you're eating with others, remember to convey your thanks. Express your gratitude for the meal, the company, and the shared experience. This shared show of thanks reinforces the pleasant mood around the table.

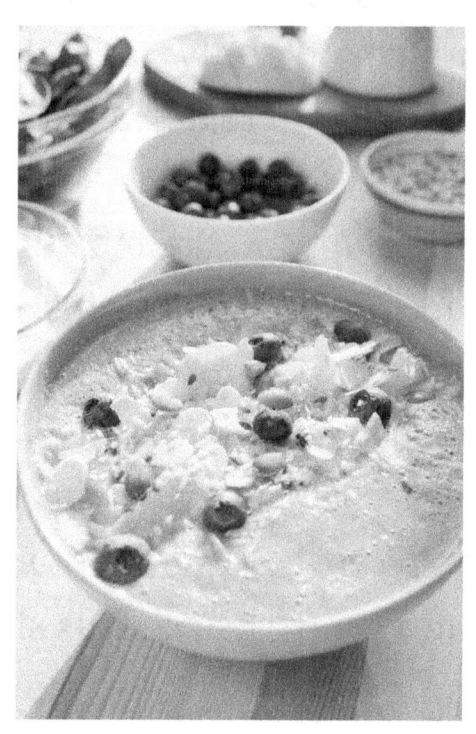

Conclusion

Take a minute to appreciate your successes. Whether it's integrating heart-healthy foods into your diet, adopting mindful eating habits, or finding the pleasure of feeding your body, each step is a win. Recognize that heart-healthy living does not involve huge changes but rather a consistent commitment to making smart choices. Accepting these adjustments progressively converts them into necessary components of your existence. Celebrate the tiny successes along the way. Every conscious action, from picking nutrient-dense goods to enjoying thoughtful meals, adds to your overall well-being. You've gone into the area of nutritional awareness, recognizing the relevance of essential nutrients, the influence of a well-balanced diet, and the capacity to make informed alternatives. With this information, you'll be able to make better educated decisions concerning your heart. Mindful eating has grown into a compass that leads you through the culinary environment. These caring behaviors have woven themselves into the fabric of your everyday life, whether it's savoring tastes, expressing thanks, or accepting portion management. The heart-healthy recipes given are more than simply a collection of meals; they are an invitation to discover the delightful junction of flavor and well-being. From invigorating breakfasts to exquisite sweets, each meal pays attention to the wealth of healthy options that promote good heart health. Remember that consistency is crucial as you progress. Accept the ebb and flow of life, adjusting heart-healthy routines to changing circumstances. Your journey is changeable, and each day gives you a chance to renew your commitment to well-being. Consider integrating happy movement into your regular routine. Physical exercise, whether it's a brisk stroll, yoga, or dancing, improves not only your cardiovascular health but also your sensation of energy and happiness. Recognize that your heart health is intricately tied to your total well-being. Take care of your mental and emotional health, build healthy connections, and emphasize self-care. Take with you the knowledge, techniques, and tastes that have enhanced your trip as you close the pages of this heart-healthy guidebook. Allow thankfulness to accompany you—for the food on your plate, the thumping of your heart, and the purposeful decisions that create your journey. This is not a farewell but rather a starting step toward a future in which heart-healthy living is not a goal but a way of life. May your heart continue to beat in sync with the melody of your well-cared-for existence. Onward to a future filled with strength, pleasure, and ongoing appreciation of the amazing vessel that is your heart.

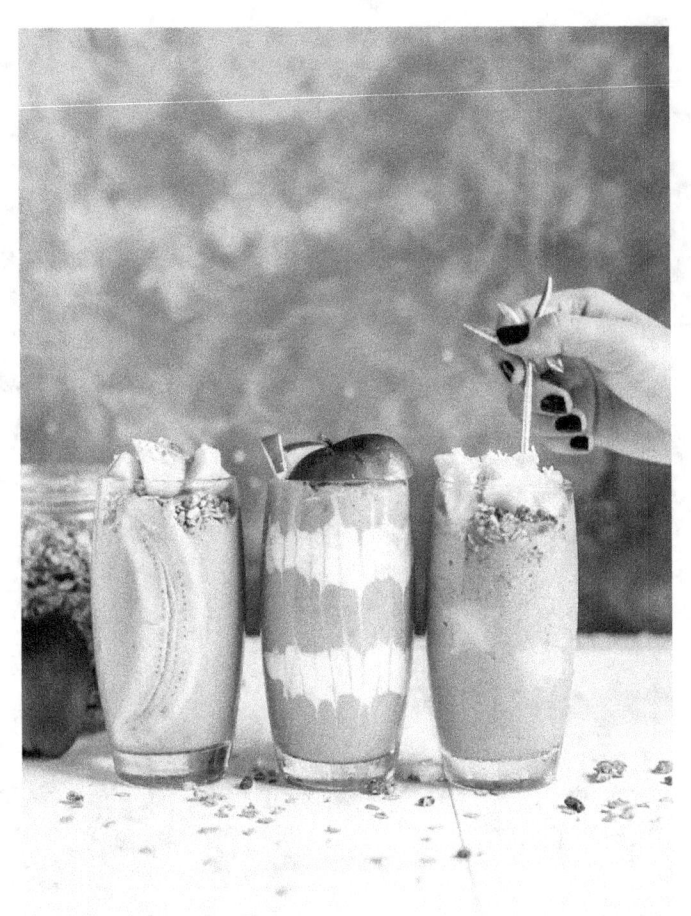

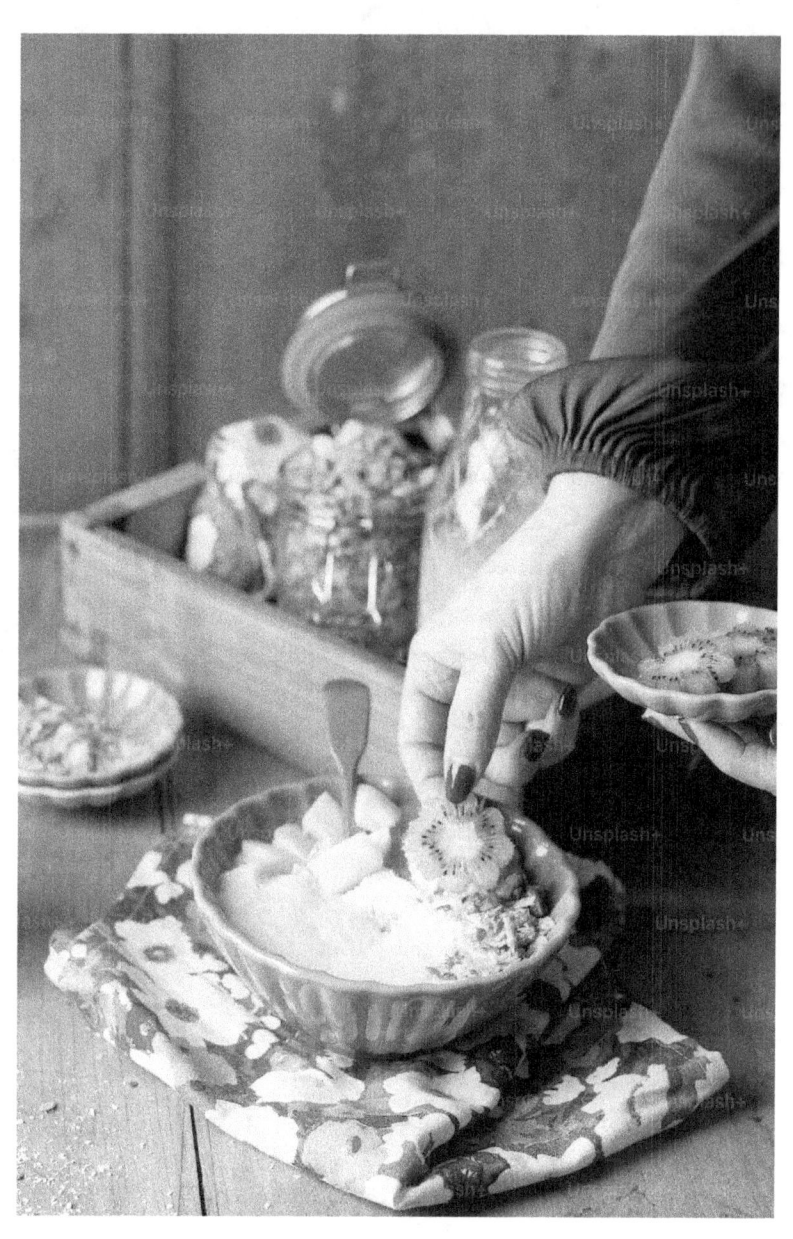

Nutritional Information for Select Recipes

Ingredients for Energizing Smoothie Bowls:

Strawberries, blueberries, and raspberries in a mixture of Greek yogurt with bananas, spinach, and almonds

Milk made from almonds

The seeds of chia

Granola

Nutritional facts (per serving):

250 calories

10g protein

45g carbohydrate

8g dietary fiber 22g

sugars Fat: 5g

1g saturated fat

5mg cholesterol

Sodium content: 80mg

Quinoa Salad with Colorful Vegetables

Ingredients:

Quinoa Tomatoes in the form of cherries

Cucumber

The red bell pepper

The red onion

Feta is a sort of cheese.

Kalamata olives and parsley (fresh)

Vinaigrette with lemon

Nutritional facts (per serving):

320 calories

12g protein

45g carbohydrate

8g dietary fiber

3g sugars

Fat 12g

4g saturated fat

15mg cholesterol

Sodium content: 350mg

Lemon-Dill Glazed Baked Salmon

Ingredients:
Fillets of salmon
Lemon Garlic with fresh dill
Yogurt with olive oil
Dijon mustard
Honey
Nutritional facts (per serving):
300 calories
25g protein
5g carbohydrate
1g dietary fiber
3g sugars
Fat: 20g
3g saturated fat
70mg cholesterol
Sodium content: 150mg

Herb-Roasted Chickpeas

Ingredients:
Chickpeas
Extra virgin olive oil
Paprika with a smoky flavor
Garlic powder with cumin, seasoned with salt and pepper
Nutritional facts (per serving):
180 calories
8g protein
25g carbs
7g dietary fiber
1 gram of sugar
Fat: 6g
1g saturated fat
0mg cholesterol
Sodium intake: 250mg

Dark Chocolate Clusters with Berries

Ingredients:
Dark chocolate Strawberries, blueberries, and raspberries
Nutritional facts (per serving):
150 calories
2g protein
20g carbs
5g dietary fiber
10g sugars
Fat: 8g
4g saturated fat
0mg cholesterol
5mg sodium

Ingredients for refreshing green tea lemonade:
Grass tea
Lemon juice, freshly squeezed mint leaves, and honey
Cubes of ice
Nutritional facts (per serving):
30 calories
0g protein
8g carbohydrate

0g dietary fiber
7g sugars
Fat: 0g
0g saturated fat
0mg cholesterol
5mg sodium

Trail Mix of Nuts and Seeds

Ingredients:
Walnuts
Almonds
Cauliflower seeds
Seeds of sunflower
Cranberries, dried
Chips in dark chocolate
Nutritional facts (per serving):
200 calories
6g protein
15g carbohydrate
3g dietary fiber
8g sugars

Fat: 14g
3g saturated fat
0mg cholesterol
5mg sodium

Greek Yogurt and Berries Parfait

Ingredients:
Yogurt from Greece
Strawberries, blueberries, and raspberries in a mixture
Granola
Honey
Nutrition Facts (per Serving):
250 calories
15g protein
35g carbohydrate
5g dietary fiber
15g sugars
Fat: 8g
2g saturated fat
10mg cholesterol
Sodium content: 50mg

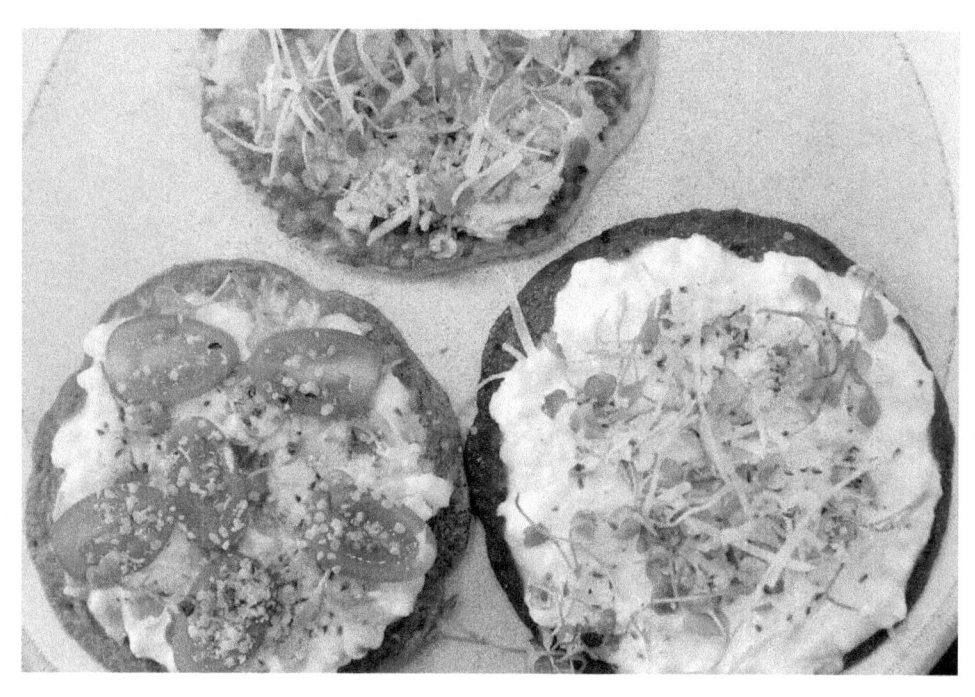